Online Nursing Education as Art and Science

Teaching, Learning, and Caring in the Virtual Setting

Lynne Zajac

Northern Kentucky University

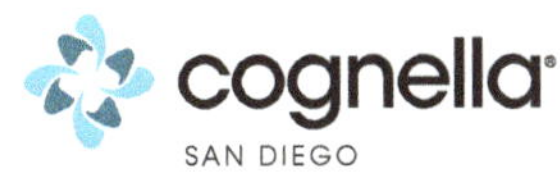
cognella
SAN DIEGO

Bassim Hamadeh, CEO and Publisher
Amanda Martin, Executive Publisher
Amy Smith, Associate Editorial Manager
Abbey Hastings, Senior Production Editor
Jess Estrella, Senior Graphic Designer
Kylie Bartolome, Licensing Specialist
Natalie Piccotti, Director of Marketing
Kassie Graves, Senior Vice President, Editorial
Alia Bales, Director, Project Editorial and Production

Printed in the United States of America.

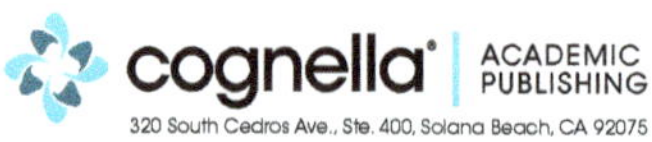

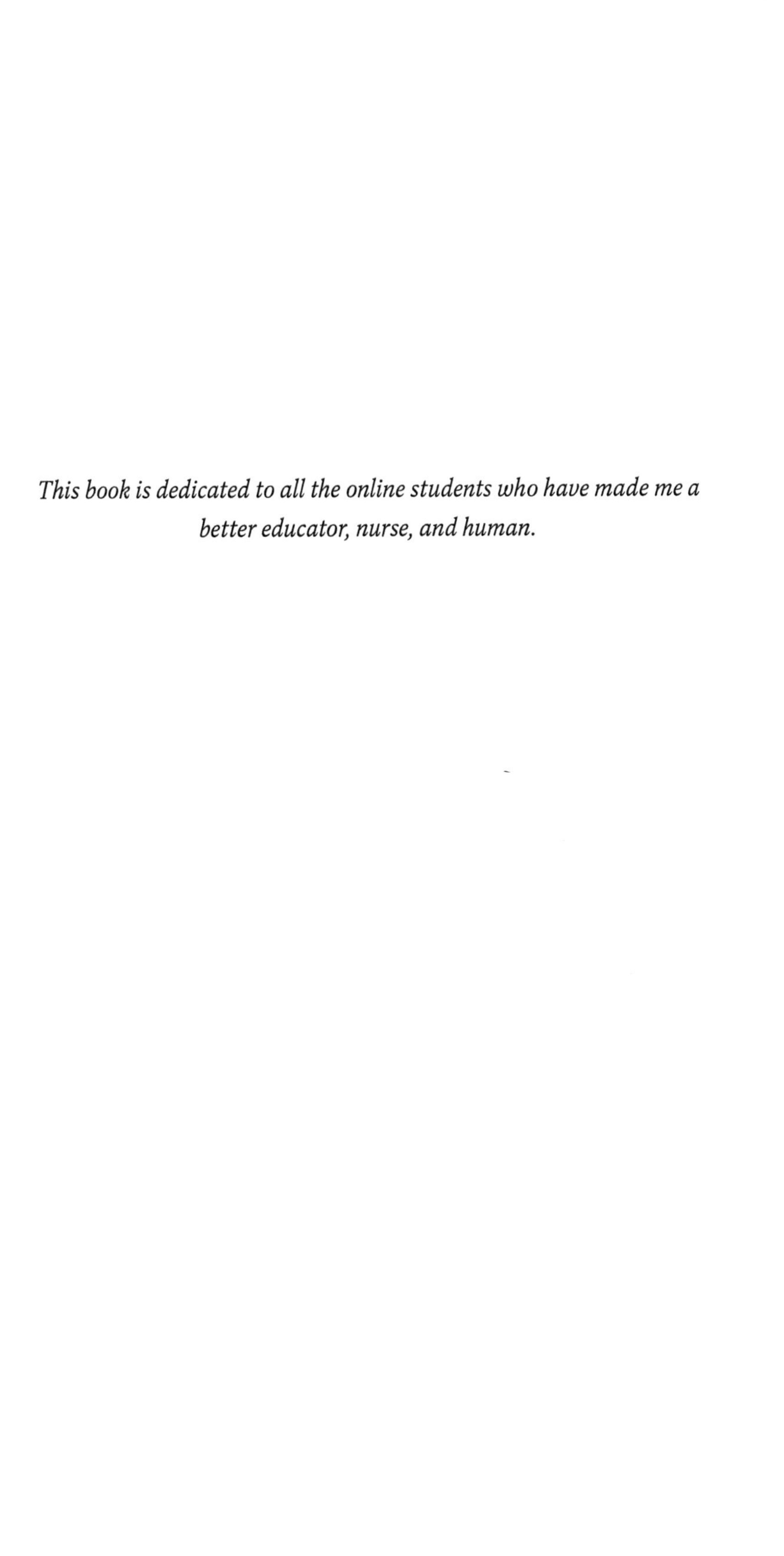

This book is dedicated to all the online students who have made me a better educator, nurse, and human.

Brief Contents

Detailed Contents

Preface

Welcome to *Online Nursing Education as Art and Science: Teaching, Learning and Caring in the Virtual World*. The purpose of this book is to provide the online nurse educator the opportunity to tap into both the art and science of educating nursing students in the online environment. Nursing is a profession that is comprised of science and art. The science of nursing is the application of evidence-based nursing actions identified through assessments and observations. The art consists of the intangibles, which are the quality pieces of nursing actions guided by the nurse's intuition or emotional power, expressed through the nurse's creative skill, and thus experienced by the patient as being cared for and cared about. This art of nursing, which translates to the human interaction of caring, is equally important between nurse educators and students. Challenges exist in demonstrating caring and faculty presence in the online educational environment due to the absence of face-to-face contact, compressed online schedules, and lack of opportunities for interactions.

This book is unique in the approach to cover key aspects of *both the science and art of online teaching-learning*. Caring, communication, and meaningful faculty-student interaction are important skills for nurse educator students to learn; the students who are future nurse educators may eventually teach nursing students at any program degree level. Caring and presence must transcend the online learning milieu. For example, as online delivery trends toward the standard for post-licensure nursing education, and online courses include clinical components, practitioner students will need to demonstrate "virtual" caring and empathy as they encounter patients in telehealth visits. In addition, hospitals have introduced the role of the virtual nurse in which care, education, decision-making, and observation occur via digital screen. All online nursing students who are learning the online faculty role require acquisition of the skills of caring, communication, and meaningful interaction from a distance in order to someday teach these virtual skills to their future students. The best way that current online faculty can teach virtual skills is to role model and provide examples of these attributes for nursing students.

Part I of the book presents the traditional "science" of online course design. It includes chapters about the history of online teaching and introduces caring in the virtual world, as well as concepts of online course development that encompass both universal and inclusive course design. In addition, Part I presents the importance of course design for consistency and navigation and the application of technology tools for online teaching-learning with a special section about online academic integrity.

Part II presents the innovative ways to foster the "art" of online education for the nurse educator, which captures human interaction. There is considerable contemporary conversation around the lost art of communication due to the digital age. Part II of the book covers topics of caring, communication, and social presence for online nursing education and virtual and telehealth nursing roles. Caring also extends to self-care, which is important for nurses learning and working in online spaces; the self-care concept is woven throughout the book, including a chapter dedicated to creating a care plan to promote wellness and resilience for the online/remote worker. Part II comprises information about how to create safe and inclusive online spaces for diverse learners. And finally, the last chapter of the book looks to the future and covers current information about artificial intelligence, merging caring and technology, and the role of nurses in the virtual milieu.

The textbook provides nurse faculty who are on a continuum of teaching experience with essential information about the art and science of educating nursing students in the online environment. Experienced nursing faculty who desire to refine their online teaching skills as well as novice nursing instructors who teach in the pre-licensure online environment will benefit from using this textbook. This textbook devoted to teaching online caring strategies supports the development of these skills.

The format and design of the book supports adult learning theory. Adult learning theory embraces the principles of self-concept, the adult learning experience, readiness to learn, orientation to learning, and motivation to learn. The objectives for each chapter focus on the student learning practical information about the essentials of teaching online. Each chapter has introductory material, followed by presentation of content, application of concepts, summary of main points, and resources and references. Select specific chapter highlights to enhance online student learning are:

1. **Teacher Tidbits** provides the learner with useful evidence-based information, suggestions, ideas, and quick tips for teaching that reinforce the content in the chapter.
2. **Show What You Know Assignment** sections, which are short answers or other assignments such as course map development, rubric building, and developing a self-care plan, provide the online learner the opportunity to apply the chapter information. The course map development is threaded throughout the book.
3. **Sharing on Caring** is an opportunity for learners to journal about how to care for their own personal health and well-being. Learners are provided with a journal format and prompted at the end of each chapter to complete entries.
4. **Glitches and Ditches** is a boxed section in several chapters that provides information about how to troubleshoot technology difficulties that the learner may encounter when designing or implementing an online course.
5. **Chapter Resources** contains online sources that the learner can click on to provide additional reading, tips, and teaching tools related to the chapter concepts.
6. **Take 5** serves as a wrap-up or summary so the learner can reflect on five key takeaway points from the chapter.

Acknowledgments

My heartfelt thanks for the work of the reviewers for the book. I appreciate their thorough review of the chapters. Their thoughtful comments and suggestions were incorporated into the final book version, which makes the book a sound educational resource for online nurse faculty. My gratitude to:

Kimberly Balko, PhD, RN
Associate Professor
School of Nursing and Allied Health
Empire State University (SUNY)
Saratoga Springs, New York

Wendy DuBose, EdD, MSN, RN, CNE
Auburn University at Montgomery
Montgomery, Alabama

Barbara M. Jackson, PhD, RN
College of Health Professions
Bellarmine University
Louisville, Kentucky

Jacqueline Michaels, PhD, RN, CNE
Associate Professor
School of Nursing and Allied Health
Empire State University (SUNY)
Saratoga Springs, New York

Jill Parsons, PhD, RN, CNE
McKendree University
Lebanon, Illinois

Justin Pascucci, DNP, RN, CNE
Assistant Professor

School of Nursing and Allied Health
SUNY Empire State University
Saratoga Springs, New York

Julie Slade, PhD, DNP, RN, CNE
Chatham University
Pittsburgh, Pennsylvania

My sincere gratitude goes to the amazing Cognella publishing team—Amanda Martin, Executive Publisher, Nursing & Health Sciences; Amy Smith, Associate Editorial Manager; Abbey Hastings, Senior Production Editor; and all the other team members—for their dedicated work and assistance to make the writing and publication of the book possible. I appreciate your support, grace, and flexibility and your ability to truly embrace caring, communication, and presence during this project.

Special thanks to my family (my village), including my partner Kathleen, daughters Kathryn and Elizabeth, sons-in-law Kevin and George, granddaughters Lily and Emmy, for your love, support, and understanding of my absences while writing. I am truly blessed with the growth of my family, including a second granddaughter on the way!

PART I

Online Nursing Education as Science

Virtual Teaching, Learning, and Caring

CHAPTER 1

History and Introduction to Online Teaching, Learning, and Caring

"Reflecting on the past, while appreciating the present, prepares us to educate for the future."

—L. ZAJAC

TERMS TO KNOW

asynchronous online course delivery: When students and the instructor participate in the course and interact with the course materials at different times.

distance education: Teaching and learning that takes place where the student (learner) and teacher are physically separated through a variety of modalities, such video, audio, and/or computer.

face-to-face or in-person learning: Learning on campus in a classroom.

hybrid course: A course that combines in-person or face-to-face learning and online learning.

online learning: Learning or participation in education using the internet; a term interchangeable with *e-learning (electronic learning)*, *web-based learning*, and *virtual learning* and sometimes used in place of *distance learning*.

massive open online courses (MOOCs): Courses enrolling large numbers of students. The courses are usually free and may be sponsored by a university or company. The courses may or may not be for academic credit. Companies may use them for certification or career advancement.

synchronous online course delivery: When students and the instructor participate in the online course at the same time, usually weekly; the teaching/learning takes place during this time.

Chapter Overview and Objectives

This first chapter provides a brief historical overview of the evolution of distance education and online learning in nursing education and related terminology. Learners are introduced to the expression "the art and science of teaching nursing" from an online education perspective, which is the premise of this text. In addition, the chapter explores the effects of the COVID-19 pandemic on online teaching and learning, as the pandemic exposed a new population of faculty and nursing students to the virtual education environment. Lastly, the chapter introduces the importance of self-care practices for the online nurse educator. Students will contribute to a self-care journal that starts with this chapter and continues through the remainder of the text.

In this chapter, the learner will:

1. Identify how past and present events shape trends in the online learning environment.
2. Define terminology associated with online learning (OL).
3. Associate the components of the art and science of nursing to online education.
4. Introduce the benefits of self-care activities for online educators and learners.

The History of Distance Education: How the Past Shapes the Present

Distance learning, also known as online learning, web-based learning, e-learning, or virtual learning, offers students the opportunity to learn in a location different from that of the faculty or teacher. Distance education

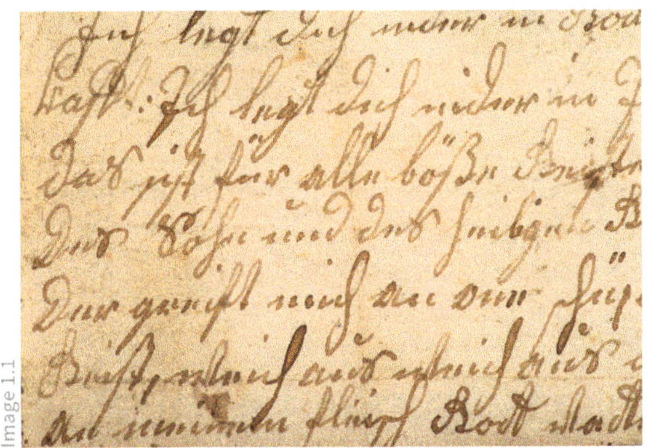

Image 1.1

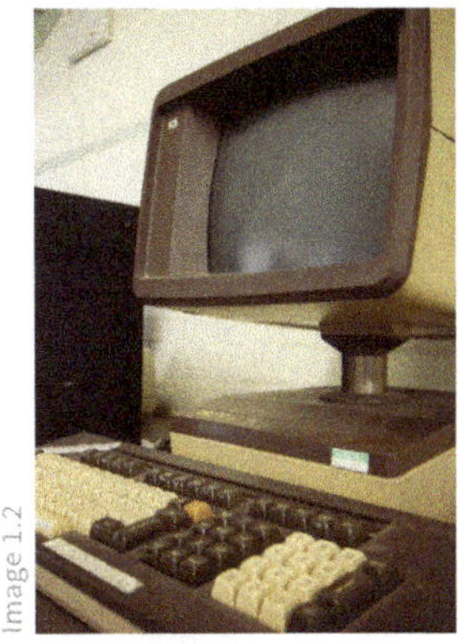

Image 1.2

originated in the 1700s in a correspondence school-like format. In the original correspondence courses, students wrote down what they learned and sent the written documents via mail or post to the educator. Over the centuries, distance learning has evolved into today's version, with millions of students engaged in virtual learning through the internet. In the fall of 2022, 53.3 percent of students in 5,776 institutions of higher learning in the United States were enrolled in distance learning courses (National Center for Education Statistics, 2022). Globally, 220 million students were enrolled in massive open online courses (MOOCs) (Shah, 2021); MOOCs are courses enrolling large numbers of students. The courses are usually free and may be sponsored by a university or company. Box 1.1 contains an abbreviated timeline of the history and evolution of distance education.

Online Nursing Education

Online nursing education started in the 1990s as the internet expanded and colleges and universities began offering degree programs online. In 1997, Duquesne University was the first to launch an online PhD in nursing program (Duquesne University, n.d.). In 2011, the Institute of Medicine (IOM) report *The Future of Nursing: Leading Change, Advancing Health* (2011) recommended that 80 percent of registered nurses (RNs) should hold a bachelor's degree in nursing by 2020. As a result of the IOM report, online RN-BSN nursing programs expanded. As of 2023, according to the American Association of Colleges of Nursing (AACN, 2023a), 650 RN-BSN programs are offered either fully or partially online.

BOX 1.1 History and Evolution of Distance Education

1700s:

- **1728:** First correspondence course in the United States; the course was started by Caleb Phillips, who placed an advertisement in the *Boston Gazette* asking to learn shorthand through weekly mailed lessons.

1800s:

- **1833:** Sir Isaac Pitman introduced correspondence courses in London, England, for learning shorthand.
- **1873**: Anna Ticknor established a correspondence school in Boston, offering courses on literature, science, art, history, French, and German.
- **1881:** In the United States, the Chautauqua Correspondence College was authorized to grant diplomas and degrees through correspondence programs, followed by the University of Chicago, and the University of Wisconsin.

1900s:

- **1922:** Pennsylvania State College (now Pennsylvania State University) provided university-sponsored radio instruction courses.
- **1950s:** The emergence of television brings televised instruction to distance education.
- **1969:** The military develops the Advanced Research Projects Agency Network (ARPANET), the precursor to the internet, laying the foundation for future advancements in online education.
- **1970s:** The University of Phoenix was established as the first virtual college in 1976.
- **1980s:** Computer-mediated communication and computer conferencing become prominent in distance education, enabling students and instructors to interact asynchronously.
- **1990s:** The internet becomes widely accessible, leading to the development of web-based learning platforms and the rise of online education. Virtual universities and online degree programs gain popularity.

2000s:

- **Early 2000s:** Learning management systems (LMSs) such as Blackboard and Moodle gain widespread adoption, providing centralized platforms for online course delivery, content management, and student interaction.

- **2008–2012:** MOOCs gain significant attention, with platforms such as Coursera, edX, and Udacity offering free online courses from prestigious universities to a global audience.
- **2010s:** Blended learning approaches, combining online and in-person instruction, become popular in educational institutions, allowing for a more personalized and flexible learning experience.

Present:

- Current advancements in technology, such as artificial intelligence (AI), virtual reality (VR), and adaptive learning systems, are transforming distance education, enabling personalized learning experiences, immersive simulations, and intelligent feedback mechanisms.

Sources: Freese, J. (2019). *University of Wisconsin history of correspondence course programs*. https://courses.dcs.wisc.edu/wp/ilinstructors/2019/07/25/a-history-of-correspondence-course-programs/; Harting, K., & Erthal, M. J. (2005). History of distance learning. *Information Technology, Learning, and Performance Journal*, *23*(1), 35–44; McGill Association of University Teachers. (n.d.). A brief history of MOOCs. *MAUT*. https://www.mcgill.ca/maut/news-current-affairs/moocs/history; Saba, F. (2013). *It started with correspondence education!* Distance-Educator.com. https://distance-educator.com/it-started-with-correspondence-education/; Tulane University School of Professional Advancement. (n.d.). *The evolution of distance learning*. https://sopa.tulane.edu/blog/evolution-distance-learning; Vox. (2015). *The internet explained*. https://www.vox.com/2014/6/16/18076282/the-internet

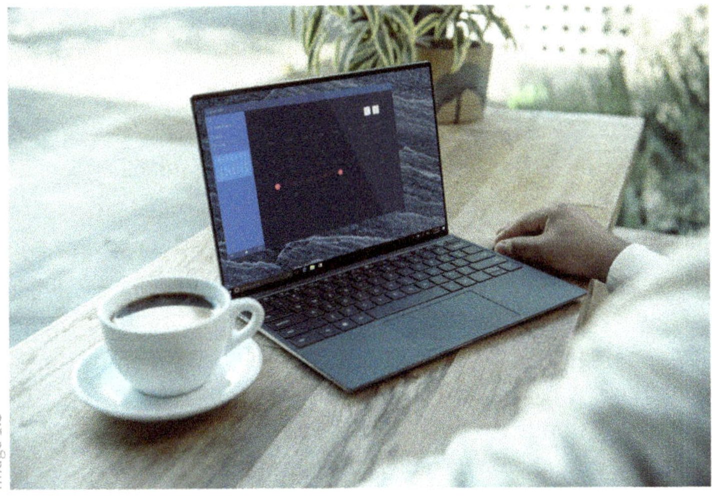

Image 1.3

In 2021, 40 percent of all graduate students were enrolled in online programs, and 50 percent of all graduate students were enrolled in at least one online course. (National Center for Education Statistics [NCES], 2022). The AACN does not list an official number of online graduate nursing programs; however, in 2023, 656 schools of nursing offered master's programs specializing in tracks such as administration, teaching, research, informatics, instruction, or advanced practice (AACN, 2021b), and each year the *US News and World Report* (2023) lists the top 125 online masters in nursing science programs (see https://www.usnews.com/education/online-education/nursing/rankings). As of 2024, 433 schools of nursing offered doctor of nursing practice (DNP) programs (AACN, 2024). In a 2022 survey by the AACN of DNP graduates, 30 percent of respondents attended DNP programs fully online and 42 percent attended hybrid programs that were at least 50 percent online (AACN, 2022). Currently, enrollments in PhD programs in nursing are on the decline (AACN, 2023b), and nursing programs at all levels are holding steady or experiencing a small decline in student enrollment (AACN, 2024).

Benefits of Online Education

Students choose online education for a variety of reasons. Online education offers students convenience and flexibility for planning around work, childcare, and family life. Compared to in-person education, the expenses for online education are lower due to decreased transportation and fuel costs. Accessibility is another factor; online learning provides education to students who are unable to attend school in person due to disability or location. Students have more control over their schedules for engaging in school work and study time when enrolled in an online course or program. Other reasons for students selecting online college are affordability, reputation of the program, short time to program completion, school and program ranking, ability to complete a thesis or capstone, ability to customize the program to meet goals, location, and family or friend recommendation (Korhonen, 2024).

Online courses are either synchronous or asynchronous. Synchronous online classes take place at the same time, usually weekly, and the students and instructor engage in the course content and course materials together. Asynchronous online classes occur so that students and faculty engage with course materials on their own at different times; however, assignments and course activities are associated with deadlines and due dates.

Challenges of Online Education

Early studies comparing learning achievement in online learning milieus to traditional face-to-face environments showed that students participating in online learning did not perform as well (Shankar et al., 2021). Per Shankar et al. (2021), these initial reports focused on online courses and programs that lacked instructor engagement, had technological challenges, and lacked institutional support for both students and faculty. Of note is that the studies were published before the COVID-19 pandemic. Today, one of the challenges of online education is that students must be self-motivated to complete coursework and meet assignment deadlines. Isolation; lack of time management skills; communication and technology issues; and personal barriers, such as learning disabilities, may also interfere with a positive online education experience (Binder, 2024).

COVID-19 and the Shift to Online Learning

Interest in the online learning environment has increased among both students and faculty since the COVID-19 pandemic, during which colleges and universities shifted from traditional face-to-face courses to online formats (Coffey, 2023; World Economic Forum, 2020).

During spring of 2020, traditional in-person nursing education programs placed courses online due to the COVID-19 pandemic. For many undergraduate nursing faculty, this was their first venture into online teaching. Faculty converted course content, activities, assignments, assessments, quizzes, and tests to an online format. Hospitals closed their doors to outsiders, so prelicensure nursing students switched from hands-on clinical activities to learning through virtual simulated lab experiences. During this time of transition, faculty satisfaction for online modalities varied depending on the amount of online training, support, and resources offered to them (Howe et al., 2021; Wilson et al., 2021). Differences in prior online teaching–learning experiences for both students and faculty accounted for variations in perceptions of the online education experience, but for students, characteristics such as faculty engagement, presence, communication, caring, and passion reflected students' motivation, which was tied to expectations for teaching effectiveness (Smith et al., 2021). In some settings, novice online faculty reported a newfound satisfaction with teaching online during the pandemic (Howe et al., 2021). Numerous articles, research studies, and stories have been published about the efforts to place face-to-face courses and programs online during the pandemic. Read the *COVID-19 Teaching Story* in Box 1.2 about one nursing school's experience. Following the pandemic, online learning experienced a resurgence, and the number of students in online courses continue to be above prepandemic numbers (NCES, 2021).

BOX 1.2 COVID-19 Teaching Story

On March 23, 2020, as COVID-19 cases surged throughout the United States, university leaders gave faculty and staff 3 days to close up their departmental offices and classrooms and switch to a virtual campus. The students remained on an extended one-week break to give faculty time to convert all "traditional" face-to-face classes to online classes. Most of the undergraduate nursing faculty were novice online educators or had no online teaching experience. With stress levels high due to an unprecedented global pandemic, the nursing faculty worked together to share knowledge, resources, wisdom, and best practices for online nursing education. Graduate nursing faculty who were already teaching online were paired up with undergraduate faculty and, through virtual meetings, mentored and assisted with the online conversion. Faculty who were users of desktop computers were issued laptops. During one of the remaining days that the campus was open, the instructional technology (IT) teams met with the undergraduate faculty to review the basics of the learning management system (LMS; see the section on LMS in the next chapter). Two members of the IT team placed themselves in each newly converted online nursing course and served as resources to assist faculty. Full curricula were placed online in just several weeks, and nursing courses that were online for the first time were delivered synchronously and virtually for the remaining Spring 2023 semester and stayed online for the following three semesters. Faculty noted that teamwork, caring, knowledge sharing, and mutual support were the key ingredients for success for this temporary venture into online teaching–learning for the undergraduate nursing program. After the pandemic, the undergraduate nursing program returned to the face-to-face format except for several courses that changed to a hybrid format.

Introduction to Art and Science of Online Teaching

Nursing is a profession that comprises science and art. The science of nursing is the application of evidence-based nursing actions identified through assessments and observations. The art consists of the intangibles, which are the quality pieces of nursing actions guided by the nurse's intuition or emotional power, expressed through the nurse's creative skill, and thus experienced by the patient as being cared for and cared about.

The Science of Online Nursing Education

When applied to education, the science ensures that the nurse educator carries the knowledge or competence needed to teach students. Furthermore, the science of teaching online comprises the tangible skills of designing courses, writing learning objectives, creating instructional materials, building rubrics, using technology, virtually fostering learner engagement, and assessing and evaluating in the virtual world. These skills are necessary competencies for online nurse educators to learn so that they can build and implement robust courses. In addition, online nurse educators must use technology to design and implement courses that are easy for students to navigate; the emphasis for the nursing student should be on learning the content rather than determining the technological navigation principles of the course. Together, these skills represent the knowledge, pedagogy, or the science of online education.

The Art of Online Nursing Education

The art of nursing in education, which comprises the human interaction of caring, is important for nurse educators and students (Sitzman & Watson, 2017). Barriers that may prevent instructor caring behaviors and faculty presence in the online educational environment include the absence of face-to-face contact and compressed online schedules. Students value faculty caring and presence in the online setting, such as frequent, meaningful communications and engagements and actions that demonstrate investment in the student (Authement & Dormire, 2020; Huber et al., 2023; Sitzman, 2010; Zajac & Lane, 2020). Within the aforementioned caring presence actions and interactions, there are important skills for nurse educators to learn; future nurse educators may eventually teach nursing students at any program degree level in the online environment.

Caring, Empathy, and the Online Environment

Caring, empathy, and presence must transcend the online learning milieu. For example, as online delivery trends toward the standard for postlicensure nursing education and online courses include clinical components, nurse practitioner-students will need to demonstrate "virtual" caring and empathy as they encounter patients in telehealth visits (Koehne, 2023). In addition, hospitals have introduced the role of the virtual nurse, whereby nursing, health care, education, decision-making, and observations all occur via a digital screen (Poirier, 2023). Online nurse educators will teach nurses learning about these positions and will have the opportunity to role model caring, empathy, and presence in the online setting, thus preparing students for their virtual roles.

In addition to online caring, communication skills, and faculty presence, nurse educators have an obligation to ensure that the online classroom is free of negative behaviors such as bias and discrimination. Creating safe and inclusive spaces for diverse learners in the online learning milieu is essential. Experts in the nursing profession call for nursing education to reflect diversity, equity, and inclusion in curricula as well as in our higher education institutions (National Academies of Sciences, Engineering, & Medicine, 2021).

Sister Simone Roach (1992) explains that human caring includes compassion and competence incorporated with confidence, conscience, and commitment. Competence aligns appropriately with the science of nursing, and compassion associates aptly with art of nursing. Both compassion and competence are essential in the delivery of online education, especially as the nurse educator provides examples and enacts these attributes for nursing students who will become online nurse educators, nurse practitioners engaged in telehealth, or virtual nurses in the practice setting. In fact, Sister Roach writes that competence without compassion is inhumane, and compassion without competence can be harmful.

Students learning the online faculty role must acquire the skills of caring, communication, meaningful interaction, and promotion of safe learning environments so that they can teach these virtual skills to their future students. Opportunities to examine the relationship of art and science in online nursing education are threaded throughout this text. Specific chapters present online strategies using both art and science as well as ideas for creating safe and inclusive learning environments.

Introduction to Self-Care for Online Nurse Educators

Caring includes the ability to care for oneself in addition to caring for others. Typically, nurse faculty balance a workload of teaching, scholarship obligations, and service activities with clinical practice hours. Tenure and promotion requirements produce additional burdens. Under these normal academic circumstances, the faculty workload is stressful. During the COVID-19 pandemic, nurse faculty reported increased stress and decreased well-being with the added responsibilities of placing all courses online (Nurse-Clark & Sockol, 2022; Sacco & Kelly, 2021). Resilience, defined as the ability to recover from difficulties, and persistence, noted as the ability to continue with something in the face of difficulty, were both higher in nurse faculty during the pandemic who previously taught online and who had professional development compared to those faculty who did not have these experiences (Nurse-Clark & Sockol, 2022).

Self-care is a necessary tool in the toolbox for online nurse educators and involves the practice of intentional nursing actions of nurturing to prevent stress and burnout. Self-care practices can also promote resilience. Online work, remote work, and "working from home" with long hours on the computer place faculty at risk for physical and mental health issues. Prolonged sitting is associated with cardiovascular and musculoskeletal health problems; working remotely can also cause feelings of isolation and other concerns. Self-care activities may decrease the risk of health issues for those who engage in online work and also strengthen resilience; in addition, self-care supports coping strategies for use when situations are challenging.

Self-care and resiliency are recognized as commitments to personal health and well-being under one of the 10 Domains for Learning as outlined by the AACN (2021a) in the advanced level of nursing education. Online nurse educators can commit to a self-care component in both graduate and undergraduate nursing curricula. In addition, online nurse faculty can role model regular self-care practices to better care for their health and well-being. One way to implement self-care is to keep a journal. Online students and faculty are encouraged to engage in the practice of journaling about self-care in the Chapter Activities at the end of this chapter. In addition, Chapter 9 presents an in-depth view of self-care and resiliency for the online teacher, virtual nurse, and learner, with ideas for a long-term plan for self-care.

Conclusion

Success in online nursing education encompasses an understanding of the past to support current and future trends in distance education. The nurse educator's understanding of the art and science of teaching nursing in the online educational setting provides a holistic approach to meeting students' learning needs in the virtual environment. Subsequent chapters of this text provide a deep dive into actions that maximize teaching and caring skills in the online environment as well as the importance of lifelong self-care for the online nurse educator.

TAKE 5

List five take-away points from Chapter 1.

What did you learn?

1.
2.
3.
4.
5.

What additional information do you need to understand the concepts?

CHAPTER ACTIVITIES

1. Locate a peer-reviewed article about the history of online nursing education. How has online education evolved in nursing? What challenges were present in early online nursing education programs?
2. Identify two reasonable, achievable self-care activities that you can engage in regularly, either daily or weekly, during this course. List the activity and the frequency. Share the activities with a person with whom you can be accountable to about your self-care plan. Keep a journal of your activities and note your feelings about engaging in the self-care activities. What are the barriers (if any) to completing the activities on a regular basis? Use the journal below or a similar format to record notes about the self-care activities.

JOURNAL EXAMPLE

Self-Care Activity 1:									
Date									
Feelings									
Barriers									
Notes									
Self-Care Activity 2:									
Date									
Feelings									
Barriers									
Notes									

3. **Share and discuss:** Share a story with the class about how COVID-19 changed your nursing practice, teaching practice,

or educational plan. Are the changes still relevant? What are your thoughts about how online educators can prepare themselves and their students for another pandemic or similar global event?

4. **Share and discuss:** Given the trend of slight declines in nursing program enrollment at all degree levels since the COVID-19 pandemic, what are your thoughts about the future of online nursing education programs? Provide an article reference to support your discussion.

REFERENCES

American Association of Colleges of Nursing. (2021a). *The essentials: Core competencies for professional nursing education.* AACN. https://www.aacnnursing.org/essentials

American Association of Colleges of Nursing. (2021b). Data spotlight: Distance education in master's nursing programs. [Press release]. https://www.aacnnursing.org/news-data/all-news/article/data-spotlight-distance-education

American Association of Colleges of Nursing. (2022). *The state of doctor of nursing practice education in 2022.* [Report]. AACN. https://www.aacnnursing.org/Portals/0/PDFs/Data/State-of-the-DNP-Summary-Report-June-2022.pdf

American Association of Colleges of Nursing. (2023a). *Degree completion programs for registered nurses: RN to master's degree and RN to baccalaureate programs.* [Fact sheet]. AACN. https://www.aacnnursing.org/news-data/fact-sheets/degree-completion-programs-for-rns

American Association of Colleges of Nursing. (2023b). *Data spotlight: A closer look at PhD in nursing program enrollment and graduations.* AACN. https://www.aacnnursing.org/news-data/all-news/article/data-spotlight-a-closer-look-at-phd-in-nursing-program-enrollment-and-graduations

American Association of Colleges of Nursing. (2024, April,15). *New AACN data points to enrollment challenges facing U.S. schools of nursing.* https://www.aacnnursing.org/news-data/all-news/article/new-aacn-data-points-to-enrollment-challenges-facing-us-schools-of-nursing

Authement, R. S., & Dormire, S. L. (2020). Introduction to the online nursing education best practices guide. *SAGE Open Nursing*, 6, 2377960820937290. https://doi.org/10.1177/2377960820937290

Binder, M. (2024). *7 top challenges with online learning for students (and solutions).* Thinkific. https://www.thinkific.com/blog/challenges-with-online-learning/

Coffey, L. (2023, August 25), *Majority of faculty prefers in-person teaching, but just barely.* InsideHigerEd. https://www.insidehighered.com/news/tech-innovation/teaching-learning/2023/08/25/report-majority-faculty-prefers-person-teaching?utm_source=Insid%E2%80%A6

Duquesne University. (n.d.). *School of nursing: School history.* [Online Catalog]. https://www.duq.edu/academics/university-catalogs/2023-2024-catalog/graduate/academic-programs/nursing/index.php

Freese, J. (2019). *University of Wisconsin history of correspondence course programs.* https://courses.dcs.wisc.edu/wp/ilinstructors/2019/07/25/a-history-of-correspondence-course-programs/

Harting, K., & Erthal, M. J. (2005). History of distance learning. *Information Technology, Learning, and Performance Journal, 23*(1), 35–44. https://www.proquest.com/docview/219815808?sourcetype=Scholarly%20Journals

Howe, D. L., Heitner, K. L., Dozier, A., & Silas, S. (2021). Health professions faculty experiences teaching online during the COVID-19 pandemic. *ABNF Journal, 32*(1), 6–11.

Huber, T., Zajac, L., O'Connell, K., Robinson, D., & Lane, A. (2023). Graduate student perceptions of nursing faculty immediacy: Caring actions for accelerated online courses. *Journal of Educators Online, 20*(3), 1–13. https://doi.org/10.9743/jeo.2023.20.3.1

Institute of Medicine Committee. (2011). *The future of nursing: Leading change, advancing health.* National Academies Press.

Koehne, K. (2023). Empathy and gratitude in telehealth. *AAACN Viewpoint, 45*(4), 12–13.

Korhonen, V. (2024, January 16). *Leading reasons for online college selection among students in the United States in 2023.* Statista. https://www.statista.com/statistics/956111/reasons-online-college-selection-students/

McGill Association of University Teachers. (n.d.). *A brief history of MOOCs.* MAUT. https://www.mcgill.ca/maut/news-current-affairs/moocs/history

National Academies of Sciences, Engineering, & Medicine. (2021). *The future of nursing 2020–2030: Charting a path to achieve health equity.* http://nap.edu/25982

National Center for Education Statistics. (2021). *Digest of education statistics: Table 311.15* https://nces.ed.gov/programs/digest/d22/tables/dt22_311.15.asp

National Center for Education Statistics. (2022). *Trend generator: Student enrollment.* https://nces.ed.gov/ipeds/TrendGenerator/app/build-table/2/42?rid=6&cid=85

Nurse-Clark, N. & Sockol, L. (2022). An exploration of resiliency among nurse educators during the COVID-19 pandemic. *Nursing Education Perspectives, 43*(5), 283–386. https://doi.org/10.1097/01.NEP.0000000000001014

Poirier, A. (2023, January 12). Trinity Health examines in-hospital virtual care model. *Grand Rapids Business Journal*, 1–3.

Roach, S. (1992). *The human act of caring: A blueprint for the health professions revised edition.* Canadian Hospital Association Press.

Saba, F. (2013) *It started with correspondence education!* Distance-Educator.com. https://distance-educator.com/it-started-with-correspondence-education/

Sacco, T. L., & Kelly, M. M. (2021). Nursing faculty experiences during the COVID-19 pandemic response. *Nursing Education Perspectives, 42*(5), 285–290. https://doi.org/10.1097/01.NEP.0000000000000843

Shah, D. (2021). By the numbers: MOOCS in 2021. *Class Central: The Report.* https://www.classcentral.com/report/mooc-stats-2021

Shankar, K., Arora, P., & Binz-Scharf, M. C. (2021). Evidence on online higher education: The promise of COVID-19 pandemic data. *Management & Labour Studies, 48*(2), 242–249. https://doi.org/10.1177/0258042X211064783

Sitzman, K. (2010). Student-preferred caring behaviors for online nursing education. *Nursing Education Perspectives, 31*(3), 172–178.

Sitzman, K., & Watson, S. (2017). *Watson's caring in the digital world.* Springer.

Smith, Y., Chen, Y.-J., & Warner-Stidham, A. (2021). Understanding online teaching effectiveness: Nursing student and faculty perspectives. *Journal of Professional Nursing, 37*(5), 785–794. http://dx.doi.org/10.1016/j.profnurs.2021.05.009

Tulane University School of Professional Advancement. (n.d.). *The evolution of distance learning.* https://sopa.tulane.edu/blog/evolution-distance-learning

Vox. (2015). *The internet explained.* https://www.vox.com/2014/6/16/18076282/the-internet

Wilson, J., Hensley, A., Culp-Roche, A., Hampton, D., Hardin-Fanning, F., Thaxton-Wiggins, A. (2021). Transitioning to teaching online during the COVID-19 pandemic. *SAGE Open Nursing, 7.* https://doi.org/10.1177/23779608211026137

World Economic Forum. (2020). *The COVID-19 pandemic has changed education forever. This is how.* https://www.weforum.org/agenda/2020/04/coronavirus-education-global-covid19-online-digital-learning

Zajac, L., & Lane, A. (2020). Student perceptions of faculty caring and social presence in online courses. *Quarterly Review of Distance Education, 21*(2), 67–78.

Credits

CHAPTER 2

Beginning Course Design for Online Teaching and Learning

"The details are not the details. They make the design."

—CHARLES EAMES

TERMS TO KNOW

alignment: The association of program outcomes and course and unit objectives.

backward design: A consecutive course development process whereby construction begins with first determining the program outcomes.

course objectives: Measurable learning goals based on the content the student learned as a result of taking the course; course and or program faculty establish the course objectives.

end-of-program learning outcome: Describes in observable and measurable terms what a student is able to do as a result of completing the program or course of study.

learning management system (LMS): A software application or web-based system that houses, manages, and distributes the materials of an educational platform. Examples include Blackboard Learn, Sakai, Moodle, and Canvas.

module: The segment or unit of course content. Faculty use modules to organize class content. Modules are ordered sequentially in the course. Each module contains all of the materials, learning activities, and assignments for the unit or course topic. This term is used interchangeably with *unit*.

nursing program accreditation: A peer review conducted by a national organization to determine if a nursing program's self-assessment of its curriculum and operating standards meets quality benchmarks.

three domains of learning: The cognitive domain, expressed as an intellectual or mental process; the affective domain, expressed as emotive processes toward learning; and the psychomotor domain, expressed as a physical demonstration of learning.

unit/module/weekly objective: A measurable learning goal to determine if the student learned the unit or weekly content in the module.

Chapter Overview and Objectives

This chapter provides the learner with information about learning management systems and course design principles, such as making connections between the course topics, the course outcomes, the unit or topic objectives, and the assignment objectives. This association between the course, unit, and assignment outcomes/objectives is the building block of course design; the construction of a course map illustrates the association. Learners ascertain how to write objectives, formulate assignments, and create rubrics for online courses. The learning management system provides the structure for the elements of online course design.

In this chapter, the learner will:

1. Recall the elements of a learning management system for online learning.
2. Discuss the association of course outcomes with unit objectives and assignment objectives.
3. Document how to write SMART learning outcomes and objectives.
4. Begin construction of a course map.
5. Create assignments to meet learning outcomes.
6. Construct rubrics for appropriate assignment assessment.

Learning Management Systems

A learning management system (LMS) is a software application or web-based platform that facilitates the management, delivery, tracking, and assessment of various educational and training programs. LMSs in higher education provide centralized and virtual environments for creating, delivering, and managing online course content. In other words, the LMS provides the structure for the elements of online course design. Select examples of LMSs used in higher education are Moodle (https://moodle.org), Canvas (https://www.instructure.com/canvas), Blackboard-Anthology (https://www.blackboard.com), Sakai (https://www.sakailms.org), D2L (https://www.d2l.com), and Google Classroom (https://classroom.google.com). Although the appearance of each LMS may look different, their components essentially operate the same way to convey the online learning environment to the student. Nurse faculty work independently or with instructional technology (IT) course designers, instructional technologists, and other university professionals to create and organize course content, including text, multimedia, quizzes, assignments, and other resources. Most LMSs have online help features that include videos and step-by-step instructions for how to set up course components. For example, Canvas has an online community of users and developers who present "how-to" guides. For more information, see the Chapter Resources at the end of this chapter for instructor guides and troubleshooting guides.

Collaboration with IT Professionals

Either faculty or instructional designers place the course in the LMS after faculty develop the objectives, content, assessments, and activities for the course. Most IT departments in higher education organizations that offer online programs house resources and references about best practices for online education on the IT website. Faculty are encouraged to use the resources and collaborate with course designers and other technology personnel for assistance with navigation, course alignment, and other features of the online teaching platform. See Table 2.1 for role descriptions of online course design and support personnel. See Chapter 4 for an in-depth discussion of collaboration with IT professionals.

TABLE 2.1 Role Descriptions for IT and Support Personnel for Online Course Design

Role	Description
Instructional technology department and administration	Builds and updates the LMS
Subject matter expert	Faculty member teaching the course; develops specific content for the online course
Instructional designer	Develops teaching–learning strategies to meet outcomes/objectives/learning goals
Media specialist (could be the instructional designers)	Has expertise on how to deliver a presentation about the course/module content
Instructional technologist (IT personnel)	Instructs on how to use specific tools
Accessibility office	Assists with course accessibility for students
Technological support	IT help desk; assists with trouble-shooting computer or LMS issues
Faculty development center/teaching learning center/office of online learning	Provides faculty development for online teaching

Introduction to Alignment and Select LMS Features

The structure of an LMS facilitates the establishment of the connections among the course objectives, module or unit objectives, and program objectives. The Commission on Collegiate Nursing Education (CCNE), the national nursing program accreditation agency of the American Association of Colleges of Nursing (AACN), expects the alignment of institutional, program, course, and unit objectives, as well as the use of applicable assignments, as part of the standards for nursing education

(CCNE, 2023; https://www.aacnnursing.org/ccne-accreditation). Other nursing program accreditation agencies with similar expectations for online nursing education programs are the Accreditation Commission for Education in Nursing (ACEN), the Commission for Nursing Education Accreditation (CNEA), the Council on Accreditation of Nurse Anesthesia Educational Programs (COA), and the American College of Nurse-Midwives Division of Accreditation (ACNM) (Nursing License Map, 2022; https://nursinglicensemap.com/nursing-degrees/nursing-accreditation). For more information on course alignment elements, see Chapter 4.

Additional LMS features include discussion forums, chatrooms, and collaboration tools to facilitate communication among learners and instructors. Other software and tools, such as content management systems (CMSs), videoconferencing, plagiarism applications, accessibility checkers, and authentication systems, enhance functionality. Security measures are in place to protect user data and ensure the integrity of the learning environment. Within the LMS, faculty can use grading applications and gradebooks to track student progress and provide feedback. Nurse faculty design online courses within the LMS using best practices for delivery of quality online education.

Designing a New Course for Online Delivery

Planning Is Essential

Every good online course design starts with a preplanning session (Box 2.1). Begin course design by thinking backward with the end in mind. Backward course design is a three-step process of program and/or course development. The three steps for program and course development originally developed by Wiggins and McTighe (2005) are (1) to identify the desired response, (2) to determine acceptable evidence, and (3) to plan the learning experiences and instruction. In other words, the steps focus on the student learning outcomes first, followed by subsequent evaluation, and then the teaching methods needed to accomplish the outcomes. Read an example of how a nurse educator program applied the backward design for curriculum revisions in the article by White and McGuire (2021) in the Chapter Resources at the end of the chapter.

The preplanning questions in Box 2.1 assist faculty in thinking about course design. The three steps of backward course design are evident in these preplanning questions.

BOX 2.1 Preplanning Questions

Tips for Writing Outcomes and Objectives

Planning session questions (in order):

1. What are the program outcomes or student learning outcomes that learners must achieve by the end of the curriculum in order to earn the nursing program degree?
2. How do your ideas for the course fit with program or curriculum outcomes?
3. What are the main ideas or areas of content for the course?
4. What is the topical outline for the course?
5. What are the course objectives?
6. Over how many weeks is the course delivered?
7. How will you divide the content into the number of weeks or units/modules?
8. What are the main unit/module topics each week?
9. What are the unit/module objectives?
10. What assignments, activities, and resources are needed to learn the content topics?
11. What are the objectives for the assignments and activities?
12. What assessment methods will you use to determine student learning?

Program Outcomes

A program outcome is the result of student learning; students should be able to demonstrate the learning of the program outcomes by the end of the curriculum. Program outcomes must be congruent with the college or university mission. Program stakeholders expect to see evidence of this congruency in the words of the program outcomes, which the nursing faculty write collaboratively. Most program outcomes start with the words, "By the end of the program, the student will…". The faculty write outcomes that are achievable and measurable. The learner and the program faculty should be able to determine that the learner has met the outcome(s) by demonstrating knowledge of the curriculum content through success in multiple courses.

Example of an end-of-program outcome for graduate nursing curriculum: At the end of the nursing program, the student will employ leadership skills with interdisciplinary teams to create meaningful change in health care and within complex healthcare delivery organizations.

Course Objectives

Course objectives are actions that measure the learning of course content. The actions are defined learning goals that are characterized as being Specific, Measurable, Attainable, Realistic, and Time-bound, in other words, SMART (O'Neill & Conzemius, 2006). SMART is simple to remember, easy to use, and reminds faculty to include the necessary components in their course objectives. Many disciplines use SMART goals or objectives in the planning of education curricula. SMART goals start with "At the end of the course/activity/module/unit, the student will...".

Example of a SMART learning objective for a graduate nursing course: At the end of the course, the student will identify how the characteristics of innovative leaders influence innovation in healthcare organizations.

This example is *specific* to the course content; *measurable* through online assignments and activities; *attainable* because it is appropriate for the graduate program level; *realistic* in the application to nursing leadership; and *time-bound,* which in this case means achievable by the end of the course. Note that the course objective aligns or connects to the program objective.

In addition to the SMART attributes, course faculty commonly write objectives for three different realms, or domains, of learning. The three domains of learning are cognitive, affective, and psychomotor. The cognitive domain is learning that is expressed as an intellectual or mental process. The affective domain is the use of attitudes, emotions, values, or feelings to reflect learning. Finally, the psychomotor domain is expressed as a physical demonstration of learning. The example SMART objective used earlier for a course objective is written for the cognitive domain. Here are two additional course objectives written for the affective and psychomotor domains.

BOX 2.2 Examples of Course Objectives for Three Learning Domains

Cognitive Domain	Affective Domain	Psychomotor Domain
At the end of the course, the student will identify how the characteristics of innovative leaders influence innovation in healthcare organizations.	At the end of the course, the student will commit to the use of characteristics of the innovative leader in healthcare organizations.	At the end of the course, the student will demonstrate actions that are congruent with the characteristics of the innovative leader in healthcare organizations.

Unit or Module Objectives

Unit (or module) objectives are actions that measure the learning of content within a course unit or module. The unit objectives should be written with the SMART attributes in mind.

Example of a SMART learning objective for a unit or module in a graduate nursing course: By the end of Unit 6, the student will list the characteristics of innovative leaders.

This example is *specific* to the course content; *measurable* through online assignments and activities; *attainable* because it is appropriate for the graduate program level; *realistic* in the application to nursing leadership and aligns with course outcomes; and *time-bound*, which in this case means achievable by the end of the unit module. Note that the unit or module objective aligns with the course objective example. Box 2.3 presents the alignment of all three example outcomes and objectives.

In addition, faculty will also write unit objectives reflective of the three learning domains. Writing objectives and outcomes takes practice; faculty can assist one another in providing guidance and support for online course design in the writing of course and unit objectives. Additional tips for writing outcomes and objectives are listed in the *Teacher Tidbits*.

BOX 2.3 Alignment of Outcomes and Objectives

Program Outcome	Course Objective	Unit/ Module Objectives
At the end of the nursing program, the student will employ leadership skills with interdisciplinary teams to create meaningful change in health care and within complex healthcare delivery organizations.	At the end of the course, the student will identify how the characteristics of innovative leaders influence innovation in healthcare organizations.	By the end of Unit 6, the student will list the characteristics of innovative leaders.

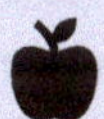

TEACHER TIDBITS FOR WRITING OUTCOMES AND OBJECTIVES

Outcomes and Objectives

Program outcomes should be:

- Specific enough to guide students through the curriculum coursework.
- Broad enough to be congruent with the higher education institution's mission.

Course or unit learning objectives should:

- Begin with a measurable action verb.
- Contain measurable and specific verbs, such as *identify*, *compare*, and *construct*, rather than vague words such as *learn*, *understand*, and *know*.
- Include the three learning domains: cognitive, affective, and psychomotor.

Resource for writing outcomes and objectives:

- Bloom's Taxonomy is a framework of learning levels with associated with action words used for writing outcomes and objectives.
- Benjamin Bloom developed the taxonomy in 1956.
- Educators and others updated the taxonomy in 2001.
- For more information about Bloom's Taxonomy, see the Chapter Resources at the end of the chapter.

Making Connections with Elements of Design

The primary elements of course design are the same for online courses as for traditional face-to-face courses; however, faculty have a greater opportunity to display how elements align using the LMS. The alignment helps students to see the relationships among the various assignments, content topics, and achievement of program outcomes necessary for earning the nursing degree. The configuration of course components starts with the end in mind. The end result or goal for any curriculum is that students engage in a collection of courses to meet the end-of-program outcomes. Faculty write objectives to indicate what students should learn by taking a specific course. Individual courses do not need to meet every end-of-program outcome, but, collectively, courses should meet all the program outcomes. These course objectives should align with the end-of-program outcomes. The course should contain activities and assignments to meet the course objectives. Each activity or assignment should have objectives associated with one or more course outcomes. This connection between end-of-program outcomes, course objectives, and assignment objectives demonstrates how content, concepts, skills, and competencies are arranged in the online course for student learning. The easiest way to establish the connections is to construct a course chart or map.

A course map provides a guide for the course so that faculty can see the relationships among the content, course activities, assessments, and course and program objectives. The course map content is easily transferred to the LMS. The LMS creates an environment for the visual alignment of these course elements and aids in fostering student understanding of the relationship between what they are learning and why.

Both students and faculty value consistency within the LMS in course design (McMullan et al., 2022). Students know how the course content connects to the big picture of program completion and an earned degree. Box 2.4 depicts 1 week or 1 unit of a course map.

BOX 2.4 Example of 1 Week or 1 Unit/Module of a Course Map

Name of course: Translation and Utilization of Evidence for Nursing Practice

Unit	**Unit 1**	**Unit 2**
Unit title/topic	Review and Appraisal of the Literature	
End-of-program outcome(s) (EPO)	EPO 3: Utilize systematic processes to appraise evidence for application to nursing practice.	
Course objective(s) (CO)	CO 1: Critically appraise nursing and healthcare literature and clinical guidelines.	
Unit objective(s) (UO) **or module objective(s)**	By the end of this unit, the student will: UO 1: Differentiate between the types of literature. UO 2: List the levels of literature evidence. UO 3: Identify the strength and quality of a variety of healthcare literature. UO 4: Appraise a variety of literature, including quantitative, qualitative, and gray literature.	

Unit	Unit 1	Unit 2
Assignment/ activity (List one or more activities for each week or unit, as appropriate. Label the unit objective that aligns with the assignment/ activity.)	Review a short video presentation about literature appraisal. (UO 3, UO 4) Read Chapters 1 through 4 in the textbook. (UO 1–4) Review articles *X*, *Y*, *Z* as examples of different types of literature/evidence. (UO 2) Appraise one research journal article and summarize. (UO 2–4) Post responses to the following question in the discussion board. (UO 1–4)	
Assessment/ evaluation (List one or more assessments for each week or unit, as appropriate. Label with the unit objective that aligns with the assessment activity.)	Graded discussion board (UO 1–4) (See discussion board rubric.) Appraisal assessment: Appraisal and summary of research journal article (see rubric). (UO 2–4)	Quiz: Review of the literature Unit 1 (OU 1–4)
High-impact practice	Add the research article appraisal and summary assessment to the ePortfolio. (UO 1–4)	

Construct a course map using the step-by-step framework! See Steps 1 through 5 to get started.

SHOW WHAT YOU KNOW ASSIGNMENT

Step-by-Step Example of How to Construct a Course Map
Directions: Use one of your course syllabi of a course you have taken or in which you are currently enrolled or are teaching as a guide to practice writing a course map for an online course. Use the step-by-step process and accompanying prompts found in Steps 1 through 5.

Step 1: Add the name of the course and list the major concepts of the course. Next, determine the number of weeks or units/modules in the course and the weekly/unit topics.

Course Map Step 1

Write the course name: ______________________________

____

List the main course concepts: ______________________________

Determine number of units/ weeks.	**Unit 1/Week 1**	**Unit 2/Week 2 (add unit columns as appropriate)**
Unit title/topic	**Write the title of the content topic.**	**Write the title of the content topic.**

Step 2: Add the program outcomes, course objectives, and unit objectives that align with the topic.

Course Map Step 2

End-of-program outcome(s) (List one or more objectives each week, as appropriate.)	Add the end-of-program outcome associated with the topic: "At the end of the program, the student will…".

Course objective(s) (List one or more objectives each week, as appropriate.)	Add the course objective(s) associated with this week's topic: "Upon completion of the course, the student will…".
Unit objectives (UO) (Write the unit objectives.)	Write the unit or weekly objective associated with the topic: "At the end of the unit, the student will…".

Step 3: Add the assignment activities and assignment objectives.

Course Map Step 3

Assignment activity (List one or more activities for each week or module unit, as appropriate. Label the unit objective that aligns with the assignment/activity.)	Write the specific course assignment activity or activities for each week in the topic/unit column and label with the appropriate unit objective(s).

Step 4: Add the assessment associated with the weekly topic.

Course Map Step 4

Assessment activity (List one or more assessments for each week or unit, as appropriate.)	Write the assessment activity associated with the topic and label it with the unit objective associated with the activity.

Step 5: Add any high-impact practices (see topic later in this chapter).

Course Map Step 5

High-impact practices	Add any high-impact practices (e.g., practicum, clinical, capstone projects, collaborative work, ePortfolios). Add the associated objective. For more information see: **https://www.aacu.org/trending-topics/high-impact**

Creating Course Assignments, Activities, and Assessments for Online Learning

A wide range of assignments and activities appropriate for the online learning environment for nursing programs is available. The course and unit activities and assignments should align with the unit and course topics and assist the student in meeting unit, course, and program objectives. As part of the online learning environment, the terms *course activity, assignment*, and *assessment* have specific definitions.

Course Activity

A *course activity* familiarizes the student with the course content or topic information. The teaching strategies for the activities may vary but must align with the adult learning theories appropriate for online education. Adult online learning reflects a combination of self-directed, social, and interactive activities. Yarborough (2018) applies the adult learning theories of John Watson (behaviorism), Lev Vygotsky (social development), Jack Mezirow (critical reflection), and John Dirkx (*Nurturing the Soul in Adult Learning*) for the foundation of online course design. Key principles of online learning theories are that (1) online learning reveals a change in behavior, (2) comprises an adult learning experience, (3) encompasses learner engagement and reflection, (4) emphasizes the social aspects of learning and motivation to learn, (5) results in the creation of new meaning, and (6) can be an emotive process (Yarbrough, 2018). A comprehensive discussion of general adult learning theories is beyond the scope of this text.

Course activities promote passive actions, such as reading and listening, as well as active learner engagement in the online environment. Examples of passive course activities appropriate for online student learning include, but are not limited to, engagement in textbook, blog, and article reading; watching and listening to online videos, podcasts, vodcasts, vlogs, and lecture presentations; and review of web-based resources and other online materials. Examples of active engagement with online activities include audience-response exercises, student-led presentations, debates, games, group projects, ePortfolios, reflective journaling, posters, video creation, writing exercises, storytelling, and interactions through discussion boards. In particular, the use of the discussion board has evolved as an online interactive tool. Grant (2022) describes the use of the discussion board to incorporate competencies such as community building, exploration of current events, making connections with the real world, and challenging students to think beyond typical (course) examples to promote critical thinking. The use of the discussion board as an interactive strategy is manifested in how the faculty construct the questions and activities (Fowler, 2023).

Online nursing programs are changing to competency-based education formats based on the new standards outlined by the AACN (2021). The standards, known as the AACN Essentials, are divided into 10 domains that include competencies for practice across practice settings; the domains are further separated into competencies necessary for entry-level practice and competencies required for advanced nursing practice (AACN, 2021). Faculty must revise online course activities and assignment strategies to align with the competency-based education principles (Fowler, 2023). Opportunities are available for faculty creativity to support learner engagement and to demonstrate the required competencies when developing online activities. Future chapters present additional information on the topic of creative course activities along with suggestions to promote student and faculty engagement.

Course Assignment

A *course assignment* also familiarizes the student with the course or topic information but also provides an opportunity for the student to practice and apply the content. Assignment examples are similar to activity examples; however, the student has a due date or timeline to submit evidence of assignment completion. The LMS has a mechanism for the student's assignment submission; the assignment submission feature marks the submitted assignment with a date and time stamp. The faculty member may also choose to record a required, ungraded, submitted assignment as "completed" in the gradebook within the LMS. A graded assignment is a form of assessment, as discussed later in the chapter.

High-Impact Practices

The idea of high-impact practices (HIPs) in higher education has been around for more than a decade. HIPs incorporate 11 areas that were originally developed for face-to-face learning: first-year seminars, learning communities, common intellectual experiences, undergraduate research, capstone courses, diversity/global learning, collaborative learning, ePortfolios, writing-intensive courses, service learning, and internships (Kuh, 2008). HIPs are geared toward creating the best, most engaging assignment for the student to grasp the content. HIPs also use active learning ideas and support quality interaction between the faculty and student. HIPs may lead to better student outcomes, especially for students who have been underserved in higher education (AACU, 2023; Van Lanen, n.d.), and they can be adapted to the online environment (Linder & Mattison Hayes, 2018). HIPs such as e-service-learning assignments, ePortfolios, internships, practicums, engaging writing activities, research and capstone projects, and placement of students in learning communities are all appropriate for adaptation to online education. Discussion board assignments can be targeted for high impact when students are directed to interact using case studies, storytelling, videos, and small group work (Fowler, 2023; Winger, 2021). Specifically, faculty can create high-impact discussion boards by asking students to respond to questions using audio or video in place of text, to develop a unique or creative answer in response to a hypothetical situation, to respond using one or more of the higher Bloom's Taxonomy cognitive processes, to separate into smaller discussion boards to encourage greater interaction, and to respond to faculty-created case scenarios (Winger, 2021).

Assessments

Assessments are graded assignments that evaluate student learning. Faculty use assessments to measure the learning of the weekly topic or several weeks of content or the entire course, such as an online final course examination. Examples of online assessments include the assignments previously listed as well as tests, quizzes, graded essays, papers, presentations, posters, discussion board submissions, group projects, and other projects graded by faculty. The assessments should align with the unit and course objectives. Review the examples under course activities, assignments, and assessments in the course map in Box 2.4. Can you think of activities, assignments, and assessments appropriate for online courses in addition to those listed in Box 2.4?

Here are some ideas for activities, assignments, and assessments:

1. Discussion board: Ask students to locate a health-related website that aligns with the weekly topic. Have students evaluate the website for quality; ask a question that uses the application of the website information to the student's clinical/practicum experience; or ask the student's perspective on the use of the information, for example, for patient education.
2. In place of a short written essay, ask the student to answer several questions on a nursing policy topic. Have the student meet with faculty via videoconference and answer the questions orally with support from the literature, or have the student record the response and post it to the discussion board.
3. Ask students to create a professional poster, submit it online, and have the students critique their peers' work using established review criteria.
4. Simulate a telehealth visit that focuses on nursing assessment.

Creating Rubrics for Online Assessments

The use of rubrics benefits both students and faculty. A rubric is the assignment blueprint for both students and faculty to follow to ensure that the completed assignment reflects the required elements (Box 2.5). The faculty member creates the rubric, incorporating course outcomes, the unit and assignment objectives, the value of the assignment toward the final grade, and the appropriateness of the assignment for an online environment. The student uses the rubric to understand the details and content of the assignment and the number of points that are assigned to each section of the assignment. The rubric can also be used as a checklist to ensure that the completed assignment includes all of the required elements. Faculty may choose any number of sections based on the requirements of the assignment and any point range for the different sections of the rubric. The faculty member uses the rubric as a grading tool to compare the student's assignment to the requirements listed on the rubric, to provide feedback on the assignment, and to offer suggestions for areas that need improvement. See Box 2.5 for an example of an assignment rubric. Some nursing programs develop standard rubrics for the discussion board, writing assignments, and presentations for consistency of grading throughout the curriculum, such as the example in Box 2.6.

BOX 2.5 Example Rubric for a Graduate Leadership Course

The Assignment: What you will do.

You will identify a system problem in your healthcare organization and then provide strategies for solutions to the problem from a leadership perspective. Please summarize the problem and the solutions into a 5- to 10-minute oral presentation. This perspective should be from a leadership position higher than your current position if you are in a leadership position. Include evidence of research of concepts and references about the leadership issue from your text, the literature, and course resources. Choose three to five excellent references to support the oral presentation. Upload an APA-formatted list of the references. Please see the specific rubric details for the required assignment elements. This assignment and rubric align with Course Objectives 1 and 3, and Unit 4 Objectives 1, 2, and 4. Faculty will schedule your online presentation for you. Please reach out to your faculty if you have questions. Looking forward to seeing your live virtual presentation!

Content Category					Points Earned
Organization & Challenge	**25–30 points**	**15–24 points**	**5–14 points**	**0–4 points**	
Healthcare Organization 1. Provide a brief overview of the organization; include type, mission, vision, population served, and employee/leadership structure, if appropriate. **Challenge** 2. Describe a current or anticipated system problem or challenge in the organization. 3. *Briefly* describe how the current leaders manage the challenges and successes within the organization. Reference concepts as appropriate. 4. Discuss the leadership and employee reaction to challenges (if known). How does the leadership in the organization react and adapt to these challenges?	Presents required elements with complete, accurate, concise information. The oral presentation is succinct, organized, and reflects a synthesis of information.	One to two key elements are missing; some elements lack complete, accurate information. The presentation is mostly succinct, organized, and reflects a synthesis of information.	Missing many key elements of content; information lacks depth and detail; presentation lacks succinctness and organization and does not reflect a synthesis of information.	Lacks most or all of the required elements. No synthesis of key concepts or information.	/30

Leadership Solutions/ Recommendations	36–40 points	25–35 points	9–24 points	0–8 points	
1. What recommendations do you have to manage this challenge (or challenges) in your organization? Include concepts about leadership from your text, the literature, , the class discussion, and the book presentations. 2. What recommendations do you have to initiate innovative change to manage the challenge(s) faced by your organization?	Presents required elements with complete, accurate, concise information. The oral presentation is succinct, organized, and reflects a synthesis of information.	One to two key elements are missing; some elements lack complete, accurate information. The presentation is mostly succinct, organized, and reflects synthesis of information. Recommendations lack support from the literature, texts, etc.	Key elements of content; information lacks depth and detail; presentation lacks succinctness, organization, and does not reflect a synthesis of information.	Content is missing; no synthesis of the key concepts.	/40

Presentation Demeanor	**10 points**	**8 points**	**4 points**	**0 points**	
Speaks clearly, makes eye contact with audience/faculty as appropriate if on video, delivers speech with ease, speech is understandable, appropriate demeanor, professionally dressed.	Engages audience/faculty, fluid, clear delivery, uses different approach other than simply reading notes; professionally dressed.	Clear and understandable, establishes eye contact most of the time, uses limited delivery techniques.	Not clear, uses notes most of the time, hard to follow, not understandable.	Reads notes, does not know material, no contact with audience.	/10
Use of Time	**5 points**			**0 points**	
Speech/presentation is within 5–10 minutes.	Within 5–10 minutes			Under or over the time limit	/5

References: Use and Submission	15 points	8 points	4 points	0 points	
1. Effective use of concepts from textbook and or other course resources. 2. Effective use of the healthcare organization's sources such as mission/vision and values. 3. Effective use of quality articles or leadership sources/professional organizations (three to five sources).	Uses sources effectively, limited use of direct quotes (no more than two), meets reference requirements for assignment, reference list is in correct format, uploads reference list one day before presentation.	Appropriate sources and documentation, may have minimal errors on references list with too few or too many references as required for the assignment, uploads reference list before speech.	Some quotes not integrated smoothly into speech, overuse of direct quotes, incorrect format, multiple APA errors on reference list, speech material weakly supported by references, uploads reference list late.	Quotes are not well integrated into speech, significant errors on reference list, material not supported by references. reference list missing or uploaded late.	/15

4. Uploads reference list one day before presentation.	
TOTAL POINTS	**/100**
FACULTY COMMENTS, SUGGESTIONS, AND FEEDBACK:	

BOX 2.6 Example of Standard Rubric for Graduate Nursing Program Curriculum

Rubric for Online Discussion Board

Criteria and Points: Contribution, Quality, and Format.			**Student Points**
Posts and responds according to the course timeline. Prepared as evident by information synthesis, informed statements, and opinions supported by the assigned readings. Shares outside literature appropriate to the topic and discussion. Cites literature within the body of the text. Addresses questions to the group. Listens and supports peers and instructor in the discussion board setting. Cites literature in APA reference list format.	May be inconsistent in responses or delayed in response to others. Demonstrates some preparation and superficially addresses topic. Makes broad statements; may ask questions. Brings outside materials to class but may lack appropriateness. Most of the time listens to and supports the work of peers. Minimal APA formatting errors in citations and references.	Late first post; delayed or no response to peers. Demonstrates lack of preparation or is off the topic. Provides unsubstantiated opinions. Lacks inclusion of outside literature or materials. Does not listen to or support peers.	
5 points	**2–4 points**	**0–1 points**	

Criteria and Points: Assessment and Critical Analysis			Student Points
Provides thorough assessment and analysis of the assigned reading, outside literature, and module activities. Forms sound and appropriate conclusions. Facilitates discussion and engagement with students and instructor. Brings new ideas to the group supported by the literature. **5 Points**	Assessment and analysis may be weak. Provides superficial conclusions or judgment of the presented material. Posts may not represent assigned reading or activities. Lacks new or different insight into the topic. Responses may lack appropriate support of the literature. **2–4 Points**	Unsatisfactory assessment and analysis of the material. Lacks conclusion or judgment about the material. Little or no support from outside materials. Lack of new ideas. Weak or no responses. Lacks contribution to the group discussion or ideas. **0–1 Points**	
POINT TOTAL			/10

Building a Rubric

Considerations for rubric development include the type of assessment, learning outcome achievement, the course and faculty standards, and course difficulty. A rubric for the online environment has specific features and includes the final directions for a student to complete an assignment/assessment. To get started, review the principles for building a rubric in Box 2.7, then answer the following questions. Can you identify the principles listed in Box 2.7 below within the example rubric in Box 2.5? Is anything missing? Do items need to be clarified or simplified? If you were the student, would you understand the expectation for the assignment?

BOX 2.7 Basic Principles of Rubric Building for Online Courses

1. Align the rubric with the assessment objectives.
2. Include all elements of the assignment into the rubric.
3. Include all required standards (e.g., formatting requirements).
4. Use understandable and measurable terms to reflect levels of achievement without being too lengthy.
5. Explain the breakdown of points, including the overall score and section scores.
6. Incorporate color and bold font where appropriate.
7. Keep the layout easy to read.
8. Consider a rubric section of application to one's job, role, success, etc.

Adapted from: Sull, E. C. (2014). Creating and using an online rubric for maximum effectiveness. *Distance Learning*, *11*(3), 45–48.

Rubrics for Quality Feedback

In addition to application as a grading tool, rubrics are used for quality feedback. Sull (2014) describes several ways that online faculty can use the rubric for quality feedback. Faculty can introduce use of the rubric during course orientation using an exemplar, explain how and why the rubric is used and how it is aligned with the course and unit objects, and note that the rubric is used for grading as well as feedback to the student. Faculty can begin the feedback by writing a positive comment to the student about the assignment. Best practices for incorporating feedback include that faculty note evidence of learning, identify strengths and areas for improvement in the assignment, and, if appropriate, discuss how the assignment applies to the work or discipline (Sull, 2014). Feedback via the rubric is key to student success in the online teaching-learning environment because it serves as a communication point between faculty and the learner. See Chapter 4 for more information about providing feedback to the learner.

Conclusion

The development of a course for online education requires knowledge of LMS elements and the connections among course activities, assignments, and assessments as well as alignment with course and unit objectives and nursing program outcomes. The LMS provides an avenue for online students to readily see the connection between their efforts at learning and success in the course. The use of the course map facilitates course development for alignment and content. The use of rubrics informs expectations for demonstrating the learning of the content of the course. Online faculty need to attend to the specific entities required for high quality online course design to support the expected learning outcomes for students.

TAKE 5

List five take-away points from Chapter 2.

What did you learn?

1.
2.
3.
4.
5.

What additional information do you need to understand the concepts? See the Chapter Resources for additional material.

CHAPTER ACTIVITIES

1. Complete the course map as directed in the "Show What You Know Assignment."
2. Answer the questions under the assignment and rubric sections.
3. Sharing on caring: Add to your journal either daily or weekly.

CHAPTER RESOURCES

Examples of LMS guides:

1. Instructure Community. (2023). *Community: Canvas instructor guides.*

   https://community.canvaslms.com/t5/Instructor-Guide/tkb-p/Instructor

   Instructure Community. (2023). *Community: Canvas troubleshooting guide.*

   https://community.canvaslms.com/t5/forums/searchpage/tab/message?advanced=false&allow_punctuation=false&q=trouble%20shooting%20guides

2. Application of backward design:

   White, A., & McGuire, B. B. (2021). Using backward course design to create the next generation of nurse educator leaders. *Journal of Continuing Education in Nursing, 52*(12), 553–557. https://doi.org/10.3928/00220124-20211108-06. See https://pubmed.ncbi.nlm.nih.gov/34870527/

3. For more information about Bloom's Taxonomy and writing learning objectives:

   What is Bloom's Taxonomy? https://bloomstaxonomy.net

What is Bloom's Digital Taxonomy? https://www.youtube.com/watch?v=fqgTBwElPzU

Writing outcomes and objectives: Purdue University: https://guides.lib.purdue.edu/c.php?g=1118684&p=8158177

4. For more information on high-impact practices in the online teaching–learning setting:

   Linder, K. E., & Mattison Hayes, C. (Eds). (2018). *High-impact practice in online education: Research and best practices*. Rutledge.

REFERENCES

American Association of Colleges and Universities. (2023). *Trending topic: High-impact practices*. https://www.aacu.org/trending-topics/high-impact

American Association Colleges of Nursing. (2021). The essentials: Core competencies for professional nursing education. https://www.aacnnursing.org/Portals/0/PDFs/Publications/Essentials-2021.pdf

American Association of Colleges of Nursing. (2023). *CCNE accreditation*. https://www.aacnnursing.org/ccne-accreditation

Blackboard. (2023). *Did you know Blackboard is now Anthology?* https://www.blackboard.com

Bloom's Taxonomy. (n.d.). *What is Bloom's taxonomy?* https://bloomstaxonomy.net/

Canvas by Instructure. (2023). https://www.instructure.com/canvas

Commission on Collegiate Nursing Education. (2023). CCNE standards and procedures. *Standards for accreditation of baccalaureate and graduate nursing programs (Amended 2018)*. https://www.aacnnursing.org/Portals/0/PDFs/CCNE/Standards-Final-2018.pdf

D2L. (2023). https://www.d2l.com

Fowler, K. (2023). Death of the discussion board: Integration of online competency-based assessment in graduate nursing programs. *Nurse Education Today, 124*, 105776. https://doi.org/10.1016/jnedt.2023.105776

Google Classroom. (2023). https://classroom.google.com

Grant, S. (2022). Not your mother's discussion board: Creating engaging discussion boards in the introductory business law course. *Journal of Legal Studies Education, 39*(2), 127–165. https://doi.org/165.10.1111/jlse.12127

Kuh, G. (2008). *High-impact educational practices: What they are, who has access to them, and why they matter.* Association of American Colleges & Universities.

Linder, K. E., & Mattison Hayes, C. (Eds.). (2018). *High-impact practice in online education: Research and best practices*. Rutledge.

McMullan, T., Williams, D. S., Lagos Ortiz, Y., & Lollar, J. (2022). Is consistency possible? Course design and delivery to meet faculty and student needs. *Current Issues in Education, 23*(3). https://doi.org/10.14507/cie.vol23iss3.2092

Moodle. (2023). https://moodle.org

Nursing License Map. (2022). *Nursing degrees & programs: Nursing school accreditation.* https://nursinglicensemap.com/nursing-degrees/nursing-accreditation/

O'Neill, J., & Conzemius, A. (2006). *The power of smart goals: Using goals to improve student learning (classroom strategies).* Solution Tree Press.

Purdue Libraries. (2023) *Impact resources for teaching and learning: Writing learning objectives.* [Research Guides]. https://guides.lib.purdue.edu/c.php?g=1118684&p=8158177#s-lg-box- 25881899

Sakai LMS. (2023). https://www.sakailms.org

Sull, E. C. (2014). Creating and using an online rubric for maximum effectiveness. *Distance Learning, 11*(3), 45–48.

Van Lanen, A. (n.d.). *High impact practices.* Lewis and Clark State College. https://www.lcsc.edu/teaching-learning/inspiration-for-teaching-and-learning/high-impact-practices

What is Bloom's Digital Taxonomy? (2021). YouTube. https://www.youtube.com/watch?v=fqgTBwElPzU

White, A., & McGuire, B. B. (2021). Using backward course design to create the next generation of nurse educator leaders. *Journal of Continuing Education in Nursing, 52*(12), 553–557. https://doi.org/10.3928/00220124-20211108-06

Wiggins, G., & McTighe, J. (2005). *Understanding by design* (2nd ed.). Association for Supervision & Curriculum Development.

Winger, A. (2021, April 1). Deepening discussion in online learning through high-impact practices. *Distance Learning, 18*(2), 35.

Yarborough, J. (2018). Adapting adult learning theory to support innovative, advanced, online learning. WVMD model. *Research in Higher Education Journal, 35*, 1–14. https://files.eric.ed.gov/fulltext/EJ1194405.pdf

Credits

Icon 2.1: Apple icon is Copyright © by Microsoft.

Icon 2.2: Owl icon is Copyright © by Microsoft.

Icon 2.3: Slate icon is Copyright © by Microsoft.

Icon 2.4: Pencil icon is Copyright © by Microsoft.

Icon 2.5: Computer icon is Copyright © by Microsoft.

CHAPTER 3

Universal and Inclusive Course Design for Online Teaching and Learning

"Thinking about design is hard, but not thinking about it can be disastrous."

—RALPH CAPLAN
(WRITER, EDITOR, AND CONSULTANT
ON AMERICAN PRODUCT DESIGN)

TERMS TO KNOW

accessibility: For online learners (for e-learning), ensures that course content is accessible and that all students can participate regardless of ability/disability.

digital accessibility tools: Devices or means to assist those with disabilities so that they can access and effectively use websites and web functions.

inclusive design: An equity-minded approach to course design that considers a student's diverse characteristics and sense of belonging.

online course navigation: The ability to move around the elements of an online course through actions such clicking, scrolling, reading, listening, and linking. Simplicity and sequencing are additional characteristics of course navigation.

universal design for learning (UDL): A structure founded on scientific understanding about how people learn that supports best practices for the education of all persons.

Chapter Overview and Objectives

This chapter provides the learner with information about universal and inclusive design principles. Learners discover strategies that are appropriate for universal design and that benefit all students. The chapter covers online materials and resources appropriate for course design and online learning. Guidelines and recommendations that represent online industry standards are presented. Materials and resources should align with the course assignments that were presented in Chapter 2. In addition, the learner will add components of universal and inclusive design to the course map.

The learner will:

1. Identify the components of universal design learning.
2. Identify components of inclusive design.
3. List appropriate materials and resources for online course development.
4. Complete the construction of the course map.

Universal Represents All Students

The word *universal* /denotes something applicable or relatable to everyone. Faculty consider the needs of all students when developing and designing online courses because learning is individually unique. Each person has a style or system for learning and incorporating information. Faculty differentiate the different learning styles and then design, create, and employ course development accordingly. Various learning theories and frameworks for learning have been developed. Kolb's theory of experiential learning, from which most learning styles are derived, is prevalent in higher education literature (Kolb & Kolb, 2005) and taps into four types of learners: divergers, assimilators, convergers, and accommodators. Each type of learner is associated with specific learning style characteristics, and faculty adapt the teaching strategies accordingly (Simple Psychology, 2023). Learning characteristics for students are similar regardless of course delivery (online versus face-to-face). In addition to learning styles, faculty structure online courses for the additional unique needs of learners, which include diversity around age, race, ethnicity and culture, gender, nontraditional learners, at-risk students, students for whom

English is not the primary language, and students with disabilities or different abilities.

Students with Different Abilities

The National Center for Education Statistics (NCES, 2021) defines a *learning disability* as "a disorder in one or more of the basic psychological processes involved in understanding or using spoken or written language that may manifest itself in an imperfect ability to listen, think, speak, read, write, spell, or do mathematical calculations." This definition encompasses a broad area of disability to be addressed by the use of professional recommendations, specific teaching strategies, and teacher actions appropriate for online learning.

The number of students with disabilities increased from 6.4 million in 2010 to 7.3 million in 2021 and continues to trend upward (NCES, 2023). These numbers represent students who self-identify, who have been identified by professionals, and/or who receive services under the Individuals with Disabilities Education Act (IDEA) (Table 3.1).

TABLE 3.1 Percentages of Learning Disabilities 2021–2022

Disability	Percentage
Specific learning disability	32
Speech or language impairment	19
Other health impairment	15
Autism	12
Development delay	7
Intellectual disability	6
Emotional disturbance	5
Multiple disabilities	2
Hearing impairment	1

(NECS, 2021)

The category "specific learning disability" comprises the largest number of people with a learning disability, and while the NECS information represents students ages 3 through 21, the /numbers indicate that faculty in higher education have a responsibility to ensure that online courses are created with universal design and with the needs of current and future college students in mind.

Universal Design for Online Learning Environment

Universal Design

Universal design (UD) is the art of creating an environment, building, program, or entity that is easy to use, friendly, accessible, creative, logical, and has worldwide appeal. The country of Ireland is an established leader in the application of UD. The Centre for Universal Design Excellence (2024), located in Ireland, is a function of the National Disability Authority and explains UD as:

> Universal Design is the design and composition of an environment so that it can be accessed, understood and used to the greatest extent possible by all people regardless of their age, size, ability or disability. An environment (or any building, product, or service in that environment) should be designed to meet the needs of all people who wish to use it. This is not a special requirement, for the benefit of only a minority of the population. It is a fundamental condition of good design. If an environment is accessible, usable, convenient and a pleasure to use, everyone benefits. By considering the diverse needs and abilities of all throughout the design process, universal design creates products, services and environments that meet peoples' needs. Simply put, universal design is good design. (Centre for Universal Design, 2024, para 1,2. https://universaldesign.ie/what-is-universal-design/)

Universal Design for Learning

Brief History of UD in the United States

Universal design for learning (UDL) is a structure founded on scientific understanding about how people learn and supports best practices for the education of all persons (CAST, 2024). CAST, the voice of UD in the United States, was originally named the Center for Applied Special Technology. It was established in 1984 by several education researchers interested in developing online technology to support learners with disabilities. Congress passed the Individuals with Disabilities Education Act (IDEA) in 1990 to provide free, accessible education to individuals with disabilities and to provide resources and support appropriate for their learning (U.S. Department of Education, n.d.). As a result of the law, CAST developed tools and support resources for education curricula and student learning and was an early adopter of UDL. CAST has evolved, and today it engages in applied research, design, and development and in building community through sharing resources and knowledge in the area of UDL, as well as advocacy for equity and access to education and educational tools. CAST includes partners from higher education, technology and publishing, government, nonprofits, foundations, and advocacy groups.

CAST UDL Guidelines

UDL supports the three components of (1) representation of information, (2) action and expression of learning, and (3) engagement—more commonly known as the what, how, and why of learning, respectively. CAST and partners developed the Universal Design Guidelines Graphic Organizer, which incorporates the three components of representation, action and expression of learning, and engagement to assist faculty in the application of ULD framework in their online courses and curricula (CAST, 2024). The guidelines are suggestions for how to operationalize learning in the educational environment in the three key areas in addition to information about how to use the UDL Guidelines Graphic Organizer. (See the Chapter Resources at the end of Chapter 3.)

More About the Three Components and the Guidelines of UDL

The three components of UDL per the CAST guidelines (2024a) are representation of information, the action and expression of learning, and engagement (2024b). The representation component encourages faculty to present the material using a variety of methods and for online students to experience the material in different ways by tapping into various learning styles. A second component is to provide several ways to promote action and expression, meaning that faculty offer various methods for learners to demonstrate their learning. The third component—representing engagement—encourages faculty to use different methods to motivate, interact, and promote student assessment and self-awareness skills. The end result is that students are expert learners who are purposeful and motivated, resourceful and knowledgeable, and strategic and goal directed, which sets them up for success. The CAST infographic in Figure 3.1 highlights the UDL guidelines organized by the three components; to see the full guidelines, visit https://udlguidelines.cast.org/.

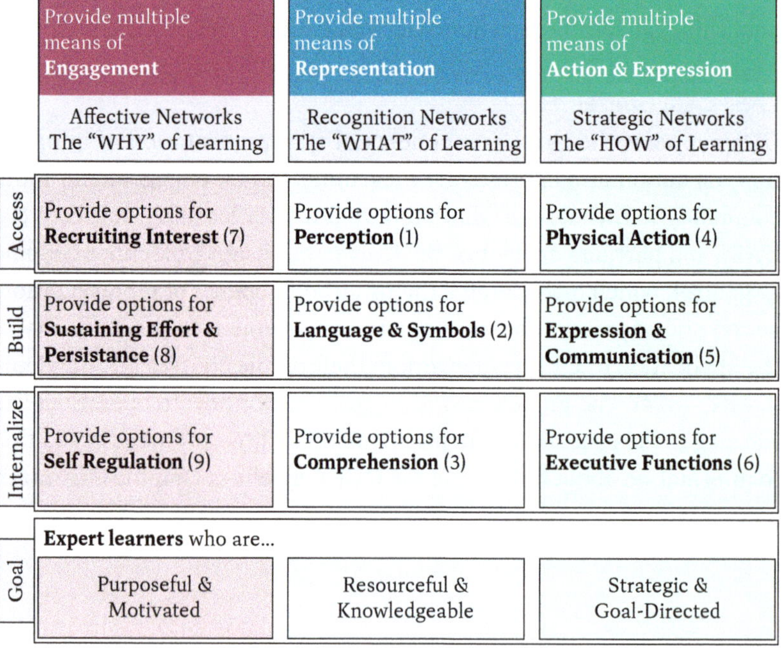

FIGURE 3.1 CAST Infographic.

The Web Accessibility Initiative

The Web Accessibility Initiative (WAI) is an international organization "committed to standards, strategies, resources, to make the web accessible to people with disabilities" (Web Accessibility Initiative, 2023, para 1). The WAI developed Web Content Accessibility Guidelines (WCAG), currently available in versions 2 and 3, which provide recommendations for how to make information more accessible on the web (e.g., text, image, and sounds) and how to structure and present information. The guidelines are beneficial for faculty engaged in online course design and follow the three principles of perceivable, operable, and understandable. The extensive guidelines provide examples of techniques to uphold the three principles as well as examples demonstrating their failure to comply. A few select examples of techniques are presented here.

Any items in an online course that are nontext (e.g., images) require a description either in text or audio format. Another example is to create captions for live and prerecorded audio and video media. Additionally, information on a course web page should be logically sequenced with descriptions for all headings and tables; these descriptions are known as alt text. Alt text is a frequently used accessibility action and is easily applied (Figure 3.2). Decorations on web pages or documents should be avoided if they have no meaning to the content, and color should not be used as the only means of communicating importance in a course. If color is used to display value—for example, in a graphic—then the meaning

Right-click the object and select **Edit Alt Text**.

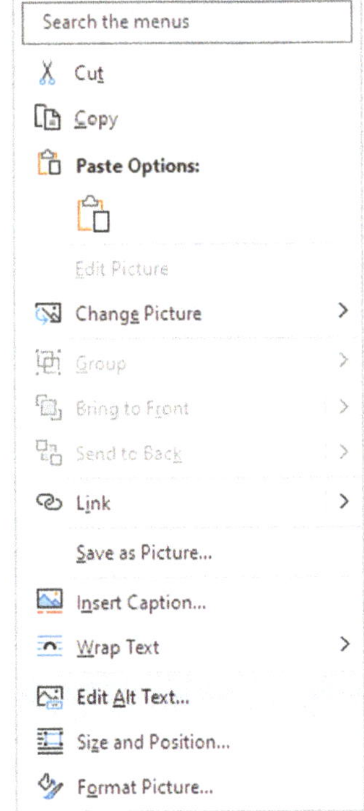

Select the objective you wish to describe and then add a few sentences to the alt text box that appears.

FIGURE 3.2 Alt Text.

must be provided in an alternative format—for example, alt text or audio. Other techniques promote navigability, such as ensuring that underlines are used for links only and that links work, are appropriate, and link to sites that also include principles of accessibility. For additional examples, see the Web Accessibility Initiative under "Course Resources."

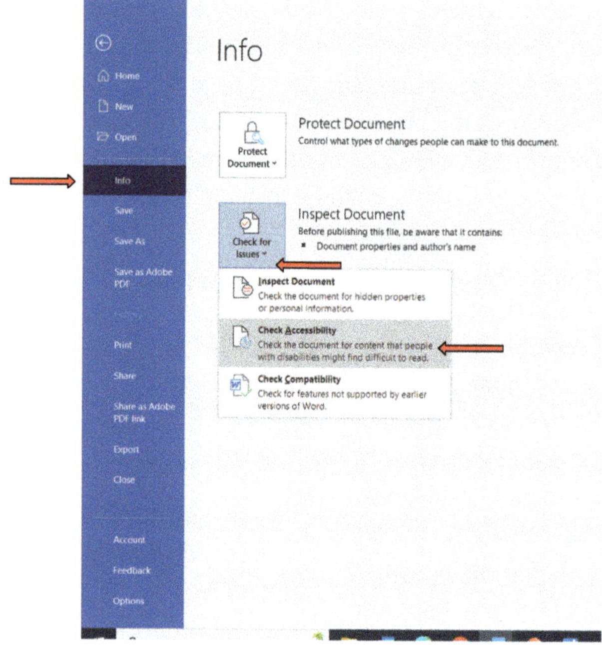

FIGURE 3.3 Word Accessibility Checker.

Microsoft Word (Figure 3.3) and PowerPoint (Figure 3.4) have built-in accessibility checkers. The accessibility checkers identify and locate accessibility issues, such as missing image descriptions, improper table and document headings, broken links, and missing captions, and offer suggestions for how to correct the problem (Figure 3.5).

Word Documents. For Word documents, select "file/choose info/check for issues/check for accessibility." The accessibility checker provides results to indicate the presence and location of problems with accessibility. Microsoft Support at www.support.microsoft.com provides step-by-step instructions for how to make documents and presentations accessible.

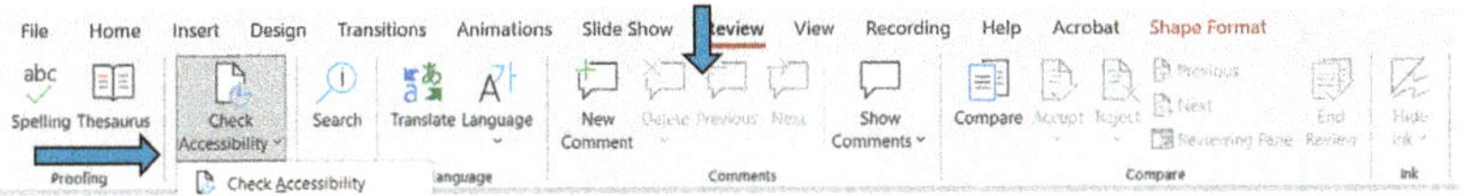

FIGURE 3.4 PowerPoint Accessibility Checker.

Click on the error/s. A "steps to fix" will pop up with directions on how to correct the error. Note that you can check accessibility as you work on the presentation.

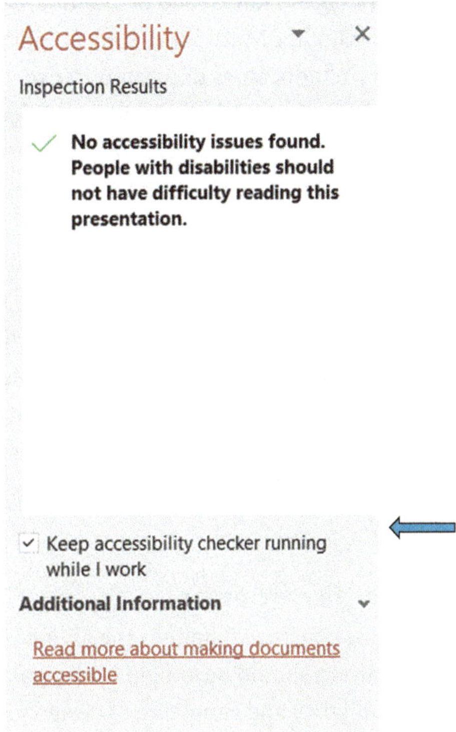

FIGURE 3.5 PowerPoint Accessibility Report.

PowerPoint. Locate the ribbon at the top of the PowerPoint presentation. Select "Review," and then select "Check Accessibility."

Assessment of Accessibility Standards for Online Courses

Learning Management Systems

Most learning management systems (LMSs) have guidelines and recommendations for ensuring accessibility. Both Instructure (Canvas) and Blackboard (Anthology) recommend the WAI's WCAG for adherence to accessibility standards for online learning. These LMSs can generate an accessibility report that details the type and location of accessibility errors in an online course, accompanied by directions for how to correct the issues.

Quality Matters

Another method for ensuring accessibility in online course design is the application of the Quality Matters (QM) rubric; one of the quality standards of the rubric is accessibility (Quality Matters, 2023a). Quality Matters is an international community of educators dedicated to excellence, consistency, and accessibility in online education and provides certification of course quality via the application of the Quality Matters Rubric through a peer-reviewed assessment process (Quality Matters, 2023b). For more information, see the Chapter Resources.

Instructional Designers

Instructional designers assist faculty with strategies to incorporate UDL into online courses. Instructional designers value faculty partnership to ensure that courses are accessible according to industry standards (Singleton et al., 2019). Within this partnership, designers can access accessibility features and make recommendations to faculty for improvements to ensure online course quality.

Simplicity and Similarity of Online Course Design

The simplicity and similarity of an online course exemplifies the action of expression and operation for UDL. Courses should be simple to navigate and user-friendly to all students. The similarity and simplicity of design for each module or unit increase the ease of online navigation of the course content for the student. Faculty may opt to use a template for the course design so that each unit looks similar in layout and functionality (Figure 3.6). The student should have an introduction to course navigation before starting the content to assist with ease of operation and course functionality. The student learns to navigate the course elements in the first unit so that the remainder of the online course becomes easy to follow. The familiarity between units ensures that students spend course time learning the content rather than the LMS technology. The same familiarity should be built into all online courses in programs or curricula. All of the courses should have a similar look and functionality, with clickable navigation buttons to move around the course. Modules or units can be accessed through the navigation list (see the left menu in Figure 3.6) or by clicking a labeled icon. When entering the module, the student will see objectives, unit content activities, readings, and links to assignments and discussion boards. LMSs may differ in how content is arranged, for example, either through the use of file folders or pages. What is important is that within a specific LMS different courses and navigations are set up similarly so that students only have to learn the landscape once and then can put their efforts toward learning the content. See Chapter 4 for additional information on course navigation.

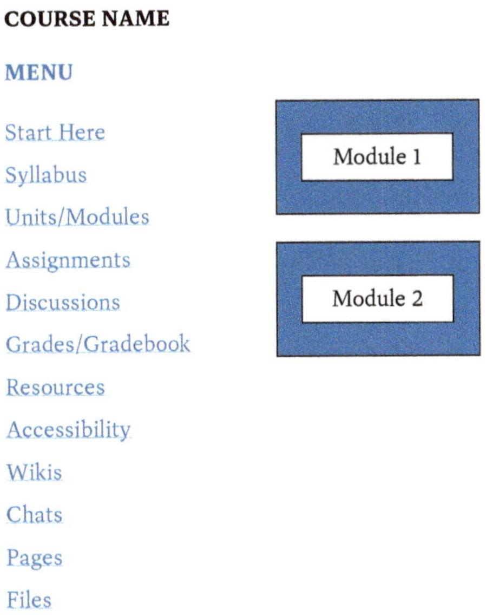

FIGURE 3.6 Example of a Consistent Course Setup.

Teaching Methods for UDL for Online Courses

Knowledge of UDL for online courses is vital to course design but pedagogy and instructional practices are equally important. Dell et al. (2015) and Lowenthal et al. (2021) offer guidance about the application of UDL principles to online courses and suggest the use of existing accessibility tools and appropriate teaching strategies. UDL benefits all learners because each person has unique needs in the educational environment. Attention to the principles of UDL from CAST and WAI as well as good instructional pedagogy will serve all students satisfactorily. Table 3.2 provides a summary of key principles along with examples of how to incorporate existing tools and modify learning strategies for UDL. Note that, although listed in the table, accessibility applications and tools for hearing, reading, navigating, scanning, and voice recognition are covered in Chapter 5.

TABLE 3.2 Summary of Key Principles and Application Examples of UDL

UDL Principles (CAST, 2018)	WAI Principles, (2023)	Application Examples	Special Considerations/Tools*
Representation	Perceivable	Backward design—create course with the end in mind, content first; use course map, then design.	Use the course map when creating content first.
		Supply background knowledge.	See discussion in Chapter 2.
		Use headings appropriately.	Turn on captions when recording.
		Provide simple and consistent navigation.*	Use color with text for key points.
		Auditory factors: Caption and describe audio and video recordings.	Use the WCAG 2.2 checklist.
		Choose simple designs for online visibility.	
		Visual factors: Use color with care; choose fonts carefully.	
		Create appropriate hyperlinks.	
		Use same principles in the syllabus as in the course.	

UDL Principles (CAST, 2018)	WAI Principles, (2023)	Application Examples	Special Considerations/Tools*
Action and expression	Operable	Use multiple media. Provide multiple means of assignment response. Model course expectations. Monitor student progress.	Screen readers and screen magnification. Braille display keyboard Speech-to-text software Spelling and grammar assist/check Use the WCAG 2.2 checklist.
Engagement	Under-standable	Choose content management system (CMS) tools carefully. Provide accessible document formats. Convert PowerPoint to HTML. If content is auditory, make it visual; if content is visual, make it auditory. Describe unusual words or abbreviations. Provide pronunciation where appropriate. Foster collaboration and community. Encourage opportunities for self-assessment.	Tools for accessibility. Use the WCAG 2.2 checklist.

Data adapted from: CAST. (2024). Universal design for learning guidelines version 2.2. [Graphic organizer]. https://udlguidelines.cast.org/; Dell, C., Dell, T., & Blackwell, T. (2015). Applying universal design for learning in online courses: Pedagogical and practical considerations. *Journal of Educators Online*, 13(20), 166–192; Lowenthal, P., Smith, C., Lomellini, A., & Greer, K. (2021). Accessible online learning: An analysis of online quality assurance frameworks. *Quarterly Review of Distance Education, 22*(2), 15–29; Web Accessibly Initiative. (2023). https://www.w3.org/WAI/WCAG22/quickref/?versions=2.1&showtechniques=121%2C124%2C131%2C141%2C148%2C244%2C333

*More information about tools is available in Chapter 5.

Inclusive Design

As the number of students enrolled in online courses in higher education has increased, with a notable jump in the number of students with disabilities, so has the number of diverse students increased (NCES, 2021). Previously listed attributes define diversity in the student population along with additional characteristics such as first generation, ethnically and racially diverse, international, varying socioeconomic levels, and different identities. Inclusive design (ID) is an equity-minded approach to course design that considers a student's diverse characteristics and sense of belonging. Therefore, knowledge of inclusive course design is vital to appropriate online course development. As with UDL, designing an online course with inclusivity in mind may benefit all students. UD and ID have similar principles. For example, Benander and Rankey (2021) suggest three principles when incorporating ID: make explanation explicit, create multiple pathways for mastery, and make recognition and value of diversity explicit; these are similar to UDL principles. Regardless of their background, students require skill development for online learning in the aforementioned areas of reading, writing, speaking, online communication (e.g., interaction, text, email, chat, etc.), and technology with respect to the diverse characteristics they bring into the online classroom. Faculty actions that support ID include, but are not limited to, ensuring student access to technology, committing to diversity and inclusion, including images and content that reflect diversity to course content, fostering faculty-to-student and student-to-student interaction, recognizing bias in self and others, creating inclusive syllabi, and connecting students to support services (Benander & Rankey, 2021; Brooks & Grady, 2022; Zajac & Benton-Lee, 2023). Details for implementing the inclusive actions are found in Chapter 7.

Inclusive Syllabi

The syllabus is the course guidebook for students. Faculty have the opportunity to develop the syllabus for online courses with inclusivity and UDL in mind (Dell et al., 2015). Helmer (2021) states that first impressions matter when it comes to relationships among the student, faculty, and the syllabus and identifies six principles as a framework (see *Teacher Tidbits*) for inclusive work in this area.

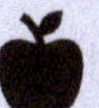

TEACHER TIDBITS FOR INCLUSIVE SYLLABUS DESIGN

Principle	Elements
Focus on student learning	Syllabus as a means of learning. Goals and objectives align with assignments, content. Words communicate support for student success. Words are motivational. Student interests, learning needs, activities, and assignments are varied. Both low- and high-stakes assessments are present. Scaffold assessment. Support student success.
Course design around big themes and essential questions	Include Short narratives of content. Start with the end—name the focus of the course. Add brief descriptions for big themes and content sections. Include thought-provoking questions.
Applica-tion of UDL principles	Add Suggestions for students to plan, prioritize, and make connections between assignments and content sections. Provide resources and acknowledge faculty role as promoting student success.
Tone and rhetoric	Use inclusive and motivating language. Avoid punishing, cold language. Choose words that are friendly, enthusiastic, respectful, and inviting. Consider the pronouns *I*, *you*, *we*, and *us* rather than *the student*.

Principle	Elements
Supportive course policies	In addition to required program and institution policies: Write policies that focus on student learning, encourage questions and faculty interaction, and promote active learning. Include a diversity and inclusion statement. Provide office hours—encourage meetings for "student-faculty hours." Write Academic dishonesty policies with the student's good intentions in mind. Build flexibility into the course for Attendance and deadlines.
Accessible design	Pay Attention to text, images, recordings, navigability, course layout, headings, tables, and descriptions. Include Policies around accessibility.

Data from: Helmer, K. (2021). Six principles of an inclusive design. In R. Kumar & B. Refaei (Eds.), *Equity and inclusion in higher education: Strategies for teaching* (pp. 19–29). University of Cincinnati Press.

SHOW WHAT YOU KNOW ASSIGNMENT

Review the course map that you began in Chapter 2. It is time to look at the map and determine how to incorporate principles of UDL and ID into the course map to ensure accessibility and inclusiveness when you place the course in the LMS.

Continuation of Course Map

Write the course name: ________________________________

____

List the main course concepts: ________________________________

____

____

____

Number of units or weeks	**Unit 1/Week 1**	**Unit 2/Week 2 (add unit columns as appropriate)**
Unit title/ topic	**Write title of content topic.**	**Write title of content topic.**
Principles of universal design	Add items related to accessibility here: Run accessibility checker for documents, presentations, web pages—provide alt text and descriptions as needed. Audio and video include caption and text capture. Provide table headings. Use links to click and connect. Avoid the use of bold and color to enhance meaning. Layout is simple and easy to navigate.	
Inclusive design	Check for inclusive language. Check tone and rhetoric of course. Adopt an inclusive syllabus—check policies, descriptions, and course requirements. (See *Teacher Tidbits.*)	

Conclusion

The development of a course for online education requires knowledge of UDL and ID. Faculty design online courses with consideration of learning styles, diversity, and accessibility. Knowledge of universal design for use of documents, presentations, recordings, and content delivery is essential for student success. Guidelines and suggestions for web accommodations, course navigation, and course design from organizations devoted to online accessibility provide faculty with best practices and industry standards. Faculty are encouraged to plan ahead through the use of the course map to address accessibility needs during the course design phase.

TAKE 5

List five take-away points from Chapter 3.

What did you learn?

1.
2.
3.
4.
5.

What additional information do you need to understand the concepts? See the Chapter Resources for additional material.

CHAPTER ACTIVITIES

1. Complete the course map for universal and inclusive /design, as directed in the "Show What You Know Assignment."
2. Sharing on Caring. Add to your journal either daily or weekly.

CHAPTER RESOURCES

1. For more information about CAST:

   UDL Graphic Organizer: https://udlguidelines.cast.org/binaries/content/assets/udlguidelines/udlg-v2-2/udlg_graphicorganizer_v2-2_numbers-no.pdf

   How to use the graphic organizer: https://udlguidelines.cast.org/more/about-graphic-organizer

2. Guidelines for UDL:

   Web Accessibility Initiative Guidelines [WAI2]: https://www.w3.org/WAI/standards-guidelines/wcag/docs/

3. Everything You Need to Know to Write Effective Alt Text: https://support.microsoft.com/en-us/office/everything-you-need-to-know-to-write-effective-alt-text-df98f884-ca3d-456c-807b-1a1fa82f5dc2

4. More information about Quality Matters:

   Quality Matters. (2023). *Helping you deliver your online promise.* https://www.qualitymatters.org/index.php/

REFERENCES

Benander, R., & Rankey, P. (2021). Designing and facilitating equitable and inclusive online courses. In R. Kumar & B. Refaei.(Eds.), *Equity and Inclusion in Higher Education: Strategies for Teaching* (pp. 41–53). University of Cincinnati Press.

Brooks, R., & Grady, S. D. (2022). Course design considerations for inclusion and representation [White paper]. Quality Matters. http://qualitymatters.org/

CAS. (2024). Universal Design for Learning Guidelines version 3.0. Retrieved from https://udlguidelines.cast.org

CAST. (2024). *About universal design for learning.* https://www.cast.org/impact/universal-design-for-learning-udl

Centre for Excellence in Universal Design. (2024). *About universal design*. https://universaldesign.ie/about-universal-design

Dell, C., Dell, T., & Blackwell, T. (2015). Applying universal design for learning in online courses: pedagogical and practical considerations. *Journal of Educators Online, 13*(20), 166–192.

Helmer, K. (2021). Six principles of an inclusive design. In R. Kumar & B. Refaei (Eds.), *Equity and inclusion in higher education: Strategies for teaching* (pp. 19–29). University of Cincinnati Press.

Instructure Community [Canvas]. (2023). *General accessibility design guidelines.* https://community.canvaslms.com/t5/Accessibility/General-Accessibility-Design-Guidelines/ba-p/252642

Instructure. (2023). *Canvas voluntary product accessibility template (VPAT).* https://www.instructure.com/products/canvas/accessibility

Kolb, A. Y., & Kolb, D. A. (2005). Learning styles and learning spaces: Enhancing experiential learning in higher education. *Academy of Management Learning, 4*(2), 193–212.

Lowenthal, P., Smith, C., Lomellini, A., & Greer, K. (2021). Accessible online learning: An analysis of online quality assurance frameworks. *Quarterly Review of Distance Education,* 22(2), 15–29.

Microsoft. (2023). *Support: Add alternative text to a shape, picture, chart, SmartArt graphic, or other object.* https://support.microsoft.com/en-us/office/add-alternative-text-to-a-shape-picture-chart-smartart-graphic-or-other-object-44989b2a-903c-4d9a-b742-6a75b451c669#PickTab=Windows

Microsoft. (2023). *Support: Make your PowerPoint presentations accessible to people with disabilities* https://support.microsoft.com/en-us/office/make-your-powerpoint-presentations-accessible-to-people-with-disabilities-6f7772b2-2f33-4bd2-8ca7-dae3b2b3ef25#bkmk_acwin

National Center for Education Statistics. (2021). *Figure 2. Undergraduate enrollment in degree-granting postsecondary institutions, by race/ethnicity and nonresident status: Fall 2010, 2019, and 2021.* [Fast Facts]. https://nces.ed.gov/fastfacts/display.asp?id=98

National Center for Education Statistics. (2023). Students with disabilities. *Condition of education.* U.S. Department of Education, Institute of Education Sciences. https://nces.ed.gov/programs/coe/indicator/cgg

National Disability Authority. (2023). *What is universal design & the seven principles?* Center for Universal Design Excellence. https://universaldesign.ie/what-is-universal-design/

Quality Matters. (2023a). *Higher-ed publisher rubric.* https://www.qualitymatters.org/qa-resources/rubric-standards/higher-ed-publisher-rubric

Quality Matters. (2023b). *Why quality matters.* https://www.qualitymatters.org/why-quality-matters/about-qm)

Simple Psychology. (2023). *Kolb's learning styles and experiential learning cycle.* https://www.simplypsychology.org/learning-kolb.html

Singleton, K., Evmenova, A., Jerome, M. K., & Clark, K. (2019). Integrating UDL strategies into the online course development process: Instructional designers' perspectives. *Online Learning, 23*(1), 206–235. https://doi-org/10.24059/olj.v23i1.1407/

U.S. Department of Education. (n.d.). IDEA: Individuals with disabilities education act. *About Idea.* https://sites.ed.gov/idea/about-idea/

Web Accessibility Initiative. (2023). *Making the web accessible.* https://www.w3.org/WAI/

Zajac, L., & Benton-Lee, J. (2023). Microaggressions: Experiences of diverse graduate nursing students in online education. *Journal of Transcultural Nursing, 34*(4), 301–309. https://doi.org/10.1177/10436596231166043

Credits

Fig. 3.1: Adapted from "The Universal Design for Learning Guidelines," http://udloncampus.cast.org/page/udl_about. Copyright © by CAST.

Fig. 3.2: Generated with Microsoft Word. Software is copyrighted © by Microsoft.

Fig. 3.3: Generated with Microsoft Word. Software is copyrighted © by Microsoft.

Fig. 3.4: Generated with Microsoft Word. Software is copyrighted © by Microsoft.

Fig. 3.5: Generated with Microsoft Word. Software is copyrighted © by Microsoft.

Icon 3.1: Apple icon is Copyright © by Microsoft.

Icon 3.2: Owl icon is Copyright © by Microsoft.

Icon 3.3: Slate icon is Copyright © by Microsoft.

Icon 3.4: Pencil icon is Copyright © by Microsoft.

Icon 3.5: Computer icon is Copyright © by Microsoft.

CHAPTER 4

Online Course Design for Consistency, Navigation, and "A Good Start"

"It's not just what it looks like and feels like. Design is how it works."

—STEVE JOBS

TERMS TO KNOW

instructional technology (IT) department: The sector of employees who are specialists in the use of technology for education; in higher education, IT is frequently associated with online education and the virtual learning environment.

netiquette: Online etiquette, which implies acceptable behavior when communicating and interacting in the online environment. Additional recommendations may include description of appropriate conduct specific to the online learning milieu.

online course hyperlink (or link): A connection between two elements in an online course.

online course/instructional designer: A person educated or experienced with instructional technology and who works with course faculty to construct and provide learning materials and course experiences for online learners.

online course navigation: *Navigation* means to follow a plan or a route; thus, online navigation is simply the process of moving around an online course through actions such clicking, scrolling, reading, listening, and linking. Simplicity and sequencing are additional characteristics of good course navigation, which translates to a quick and easy process for students.

Chapter Overview and Objectives

This chapter provides the learner with instructions on how to set up course navigation in the process of course design. Good course navigation means that the online student spends time learning content rather than spending time searching for assignments and materials. Specific elements of course navigation are actions that link to assignments, resources, and course materials; learners are encouraged to practice these course design skills. In addition, the chapter includes best practices for supporting online students to successfully (1) navigate within the course learning management system, (2) connect to university/college/instructional technology (IT) resources, and (3) use the principles of netiquette for online learning. Learners will create a mock "Start Here" module. Faculty are encouraged to use institutional and instructional resources such as online course designers as needed.

In this chapter, the learner will:

1. Examine best practices for online course navigation for students and educators.
2. Create a "Start Here" module.
3. Identify the elements of netiquette necessary for online learning.
4. Investigate university/college/program resources appropriate for placement in the online course.
5. Identify opportunities to collaborate with instructional technology and design personnel.

Principles of Navigation: Getting Around the Course

Faculty and course designers consider consistent course structure and ease of navigation as critical elements of online course design (Bollinger & Martin, 2021). Online course navigation is the student's ability to move throughout the course from one place to another, for example, from a module activity to a course assignment. In other words, navigation refers to the elements in the course that get students where they need to go. Key characteristics of navigation are that elements are easy, flexible, intuitive, organized, and fluid. Learning management systems (LMSs) contain features to facilitate appropriate course navigation, for example, element linking capabilities and a consistent, standardized structure and interface in courses and units/modules (Ralston-Berg & Braatz, 2021). The ease of navigation maximizes the students' time so that less effort is spent on course technology and searching for course components and more time is spent on learning content.

Element linking capabilities refer to the student clicking on an item and having the item open on the LMS page. Faculty create this action in the course by using the "link" feature noted by a chain icon or the "link" word found in most LMSs (Instructure, 2023; Moodle, 2023; Sakai, 2023). Faculty click on the link icon or word from a pop-up menu or tab and then add the module or assignment destination as an address or title that will then show as a hyperlink or link to students. Usually, the hyperlink shows as a word or words that are underlined in blue. This hyperlink creates a connection between two parts of the course. Students should have multiple ways to link to an item. For example, students should be able to link to a graded discussion board (DB) activity from the assignment segment of the course and also link to the same DB activity from the specific module where the DB is assigned.

One best practice for navigation is the use of a consistent standardized structure and interface; *standardized structure* means having a similar look and configuration to the element, whereas *interface* denotes interacting with the elements similarly between modules and courses (Ralston-Berg & Braatz, 2021). Students value consistency among and within courses (McMullan et al., 2021). Online courses demonstrate a consistent look using standard course items such as the "start here/begin here" section, syllabus, course introduction, modules, assignments, discussions, gradebooks, etc. These standard course items are in the same location from course to course (Figure 4.1). Item consistency is also important for the format and location of items in weekly modules or units. For example, each module should show consistency in the placement of module objectives, overview, activities, resources, and assignments. The use of a course template assists with this consistency among courses and between modules (Konstantinidis, 2022; Ralston-Berg & Braatz, 2021).

Recall the discussion in Chapter 3 and image in Figure 3.6 about the simplicity and similarity of course design. The concept of navigation factors into this simplicity by connecting components by clicking from one to another. Figure 4.1 adds additional information about course and module consistency and student navigation to Figure 3.6.

An additional method to demonstrate the connection and flow between the course and module elements is provided in the flowchart in Figure 4.3 (Ralston-Berg & Braatz, 2021), which complements the content narrative of the course map introduced in Chapter 2.

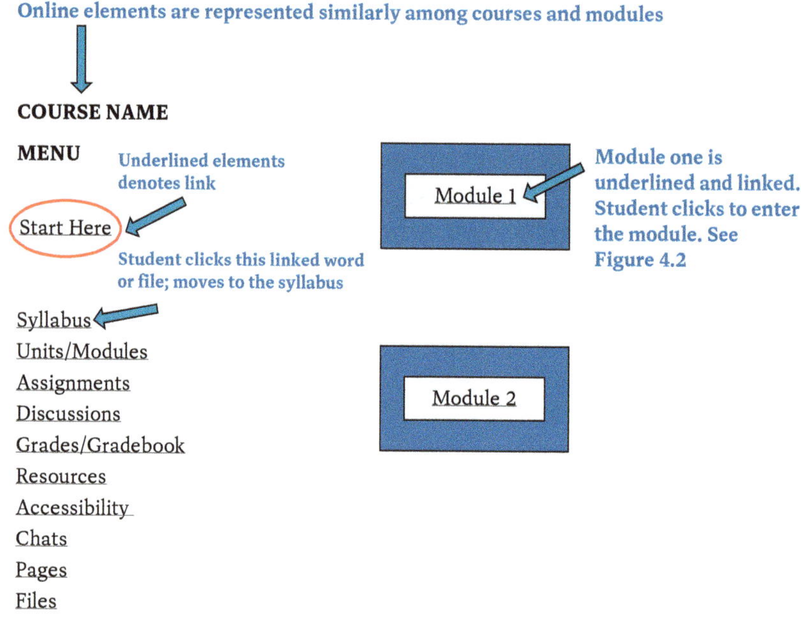

FIGURE 4.1 Examples of Course Elements in a Two-Module Course to Demonstrate a Consistent, Standardized Course Structure and Ease of Interface and Navigation.

Each module appears similarly but with different course content

MODULE ONE
Topic

Student clicks this linked word;
moves to the overview for a summary of the module expectations

Overview
Objectives
Experiences/Activities
    Assignments
    Activities
    Readings

Teaching Activities Each underline word is a link to a place in the module
    Faculty lectures
    Videos
    Module Resources
Module Wrap Up

Best practice is the use of consistent, standardized module structure and ease of interface and navigation

FIGURE 4.2 Example of Organization of Module Elements to Demonstrate a Consistent, Standardized Module Structure and Ease of Interface and Navigation.

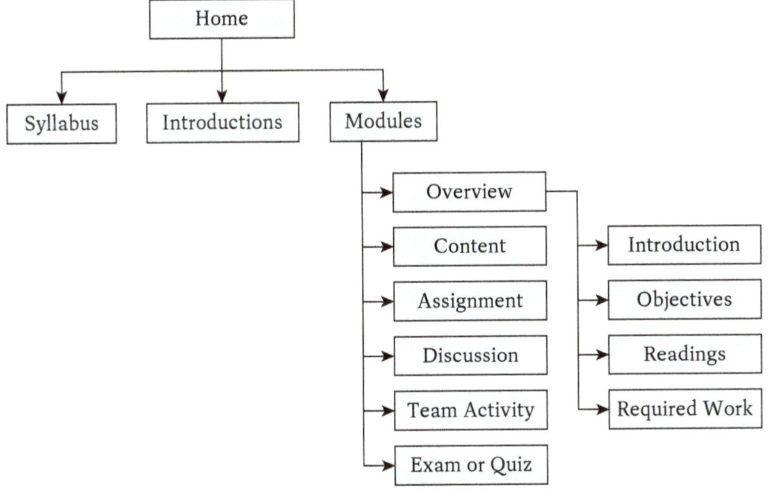

FIGURE 4.3 Flowchart to Denote Course Structure and Naming Conventions.

Contents of the Course "Start Here" Section

The "Begin Here," "Start Here," "Module 0 Area," hereby known as the "Start Here" section, introduces the online student to course policies, resources, classmates, faculty, technology requirements, and learning tools (Figure 4.4), all of which are key to course navigation and course success. This section is structured the same in all online courses in the program/curriculum, although the content varies depending on the course. These introduction activities are the first steps in engaging the students as a community of learners (Garrison et al., 2000). The effective use of the "Start Here" concept/module assists the faculty in establishing their online cognitive, teaching, and social presence (Garrison et al., 2000) and for students parallels the first day of the class experienced by a traditional in-person class (Wengier, 2022). In general, students perceive that instructor presence, feedback, and use of clear instructions are key attributes of faculty excellence in the online learning environment (Wright et al., 2023; Zajac & Lane, 2020). The use of the "Start Here" feature reinforces these attributes. A list of each of the "Start Here" components is provided in Figure 4.4.

1. From the course menu- click on Start Here

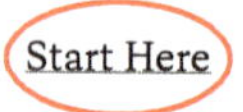

2. Suggested List of 'Start Here' components

Introduction to the course and contents
Tips for course success
Faculty Introduction
Learning Tools
Technology and Requirements
Institution/University policies/Student resources
Online etiquette
Student introductions
Link to the discussion board for student introductions

FIGURE 4.4 Components of the "Start Here" Module.

Explanation of the "Start Here" Components

Course and Content Introduction

The introduction contains a brief description of the course and/or overview of the main concepts along with the course objectives. In addition, faculty may discuss how the course aligns with others in the curriculum and/or how the content applies to the student's chosen major or discipline. Students can find tips for how to navigate the course and/or a brief outline of the course structure. A faculty-created video about the online course enhances instructor immediacy and presence (Seckman, 2018).

Tips for Online Course Success

Faculty share tips for student success in the course in this section. Examples are study suggestions, assignment preparation recommendations, time management prompts, ideas for maximizing course resources, and referral to the course Q&A discussion board. This is an opportunity for faculty to post availability and office hours and encourage students to reach out with course questions.

Faculty Introduction

The faculty introduction section highlights the instructor's character and passion for the course material (Wengier, 2022). This is the faculty's opportunity to personally welcome students to the course for immediate engagement. Faculty have the opportunity to share professional and personal information with their students, including educational experience and practical involvement with the major/discipline and course content, as well as personal interests or hobbies, etc. This section includes the faculty's contact information and includes the preferred method or the best way to reach faculty for the duration of the course. Virtual office hours are posted here. Minimally, this section can be short biographical text with a photo or photos attached. A faculty-created video enhances faculty immediacy in online courses (Seckman, 2018); the faculty could place a biographical video in this section of "Start Here." The *Teacher Tidbits* provides a sample bio that demonstrates typical biographical information as well as a personal welcome, enthusiasm for and experience with course content, personal interests, contact information, and investment in student success.

Learning Tools

This section presents the students with the main course tools used in the LMS and in the course and describes information specific to privacy and accessibility. Other examples of learning tools are video platforms such as YouTube (https://www.youtube.com), antiplagiarism tools, academic integrity tools, test administration software, and other tools used in learning and assessment activities. Steps to promote students' privacy and accessibility are addressed with each learning tool. See the Chapter Resources for examples of privacy and accessibility statements for a variety of tool sources.

TEACHER TIDBITS FOR SAMPLE FACULTY BIO/INTRODUCTION

Hello and welcome to class! My name is Lily Tims. Please call me Dr. T or Dr. Tims. I am certified as a family nurse practitioner and currently practicing one day per week in a busy pediatric office. I am so excited to share my practice experiences with you during this course. I have enjoyed teaching nursing for the past 15 years in both undergraduate and graduate programs, including face-to-face and online courses. I earned a PhD in Nursing from University X and an MSN from University Z. My areas of nursing expertise, interest, and research are pediatric growth and development, care of neurodivergent children, online education, and holistic nursing. In my spare time, I enjoy trips to museums and the beach! I have two daughters in high school and a rescue pup named Abby. My email is Ltims@myuniversity.com and my phone number is 555-555-5555. The best time to phone me is late afternoon or early evening. I check my email frequently if you prefer email. I am looking forward to meeting you! Please reach out with questions about the course. My goal is to help you succeed!

Technology and Requirements

This section informs students of the activities required on their technology devices. Minimally, students should have the capability to attach documents to email, download and upload documents, listen to and watch videos, etc. In addition, students learn what internet browsers are appropriate for the course activities. This is a good area to place the contact information for the IT department. Remind students to contact IT for glitches that may occur while navigating the course. See "Grumbles and Glitches" at the end of the chapter.

Institution/University Policies

This section links to university policies that may impact the students while enrolled in an online course. Here students should find connections to items such as the university drop/add course policy, academic dishonesty guidelines, attendance requirements, copyright laws, university disability/accessibility services, and other institution-specific procedures. This section could house an institution-specific syllabus, if applicable.

Student Resources

The section presents resources appropriate to the online student, especially if their academic program is fully online. Student resources are entities that provide academic, social, and psychological support while a learner is enrolled at the university. Each resource should link to a webpage that describes the "who, what, and when" of the resource. Examples of resources are university offices such as the registrar, financial aid, student services, veteran support programs, tutoring and writing resources, counseling centers, information technology help desk/assistance, and appropriate social activities as appropriate for an online student. Another idea is to list 24/7 resources for online students in this section as well.

Online Etiquette

This section contains rules for online communication and behavior known as online etiquette, or "netiquette," to ensure an environment conducive to learning for all students. Faculty are responsible for educating students in appropriate communication methods when using technology and holding students accountable (Mikolon et al., 2022). The virtual world has evolved so that etiquette behavior includes education about actions such as cyberbullying and plagiarism so that students remain safe in the online environment (Gupta et al., 2022). See Figure 4.5 for examples of appropriate online etiquette for writing email and posts on DBs and social media sites.

Student Introductions in the Discussion Board

Students introduce themselves in the first DB. For consistency in DB responses, faculty can set parameters and ask students for specific information to include in their introductions. Ideas for posting introductions include past experience with the course material; personal background, such as where they work and live; how many online courses they have taken; hobbies; interests; and a fun fact about themselves. The introduction activity should generate excitement as well as provide meaningful information about the student for early course engagement. Students are encouraged to post a picture of themselves if they so choose. Explain that students need only post what they feel comfortable sharing. A link from this section navigates the student to the discussion board to post their introduction.

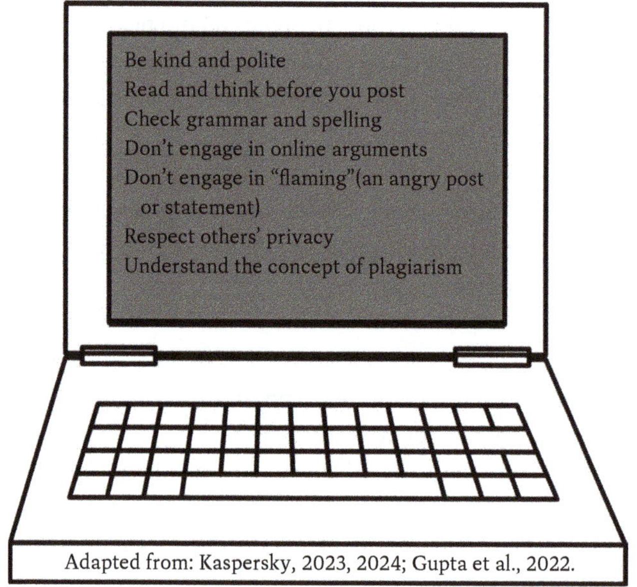

FIGURE 4.5 Example: Basic Rules for Online Etiquette (Netiquette).

The "Start Here" area is most often the first point of course exposure for the students. The area should be friendly, informative, supportive, and aid the student in navigation. Faculty choose these introductory materials to promote success in the online course. The "Start Here" area offers students an environment conducive to learning to set the student on a path for success.

SHOW WHAT YOU KNOW ASSIGNMENT

Think about an online course that you teach or my teach in the future. What items or topics would you include in the "Start Here" area in your online course? Complete the template to create a mock "Start Here" area.

Template for Start Here Module

Start Here: Category	Category Item Name—List Here
Introduction to the course and contents	Example: Brief course description or content overview; use of the content in the discipline
Faculty introduction	
Learning tools	
Technology and requirements	
Institution/university policies/ student resources	[Remember to include links here.]
Online etiquette	
Student introductions with a link to the discussion board	
Other categories?	

Use of Resources for Assistance, Collaboration, and Troubleshooting

Collaboration

Online faculty should have access to resources that are available at the institution. For example, check the university's teaching/learning center for helpful hints for designing online courses using best practices such as creating course connections and providing easy navigation for students. Teaching-learning centers have seminars, workshops, presentations, and "lunch and learn" sessions that may cover topics such as navigation, course design, and assembly. Remember that the LMS has learning guides and links to online learning communities for assistance with course design (see Chapter 2, Chapter Resources). Faculty will need specific information associated with the course design and assembly that is exclusive to their institution's particular LMS. A review of the university's policies for items such as netiquette, syllabus requirements, and use of standard templates for online course development is important for navigation.

If available at the institution, contact the IT department about collaborating with a course designer to assist with the development of course configuration and navigation. An online course/instructional designer is a person educated or experienced with instructional technology and who works with course faculty to construct and provide learning materials and course experiences for online learners. Novice and experienced online faculty are encouraged to use instructional designers, especially for a course redesign or new design. There is a learning curve associated with the rapidly changing technology and the development of new strategies for online education; instructional designers have this knowledge and are available to collaborate with faculty (Richardson et al., 2019). Online instructional designers can create learning products, analyze learning needs, assess existing course teaching materials, develop formative and summative evaluation plans, and design the course structure or flow (Jordan, 2022), which supports navigation. Recommendations to enhance collaborative efforts between faculty and designers include demonstration of respect, understanding, and support for each other's roles; mutual trust in the work; and recognition of the design work by university administrators and leaders (Richardson et al., 2019). Instructional designers and institutional resources are valuable assets to guide faculty in the development of ideas discussed in this chapter. See Chapter 2 for a review of the roles of online support personnel.

Troubleshooting Technology

Despite faculty preparation and good intentions, technological glitches occur and students will report technology issues; see the "Grumbles and Glitches." Refer students to the university technology service or IT department when glitches occur. Remember that IT contact information is located in the "Start Here" section. Faculty are not expected to be proficient in every type of portable or computer device; however, some flexibility is warranted to move assignment due dates in the event of student technology challenges.

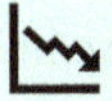

GRUMBLES AND GLITCHES: STUDENT ISSUES

1. Broken links (refer to LMS directions for fixing broken links)
2. User experience
3. Compatibility issues with phones and tablets
4. Navigation barriers
5. Inability to play audio or video recordings
6. Accessibility issues (refer student to IT for assistance)

Adapted from: Pappas, C. (2021). *E-learning industry. 7 top technical difficulties in online training and tips to get rid of the glitches.* https://elearningindustry.com/top-technical-difficulties-in-online-training-tips-get-rid-glitches

Conclusion

Online course navigation is important for students to achieve course outcomes. Similarity and consistency between courses and among modules/units along with connection to course elements promote ease of use. Students are more successful when they spend their time learning content rather than the course mechanics. Faculty can provide students with a solid foundation for the course through the use of a "Start Here" area to introduce content, policies, strategies, expectations, and resources. In addition, online faculty benefit from using university resources and instructional course designers to assist with course design and navigation. Using best practices in online course design supports student success!

TAKE 5

List five take-away points from Chapter 4.

What did you learn?

1.
2.
3.
4.
5.

What additional information do you need to understand the concepts? See the Chapter Resources for additional material.

CHAPTER ACTIVITIES

1. Complete the "Start Here" template as directed in the "Show What You Know Assignment."
2. Discussion question: Consider an online course that you are teaching or have taken that you would like to revise. What are some ways that you could foster collaboration with a course designer to ensure success with the revision?
3. Sharing on Caring: Add to your journal either daily or weekly.

CHAPTER RESOURCES

1. Additional information on netiquette:

   Kaspersky. (2023). *What is netiquette*. [Video]. YouTube. https://www.youtube.com/watch?v=CWbtbycHZok

2. Examples of policies for course tools:

   YouTube. (n.d.). *How does YouTube maintain user privacy?* https://www.youtube.com/howyoutubeworks/our-commitments/protecting-user-data/

   Turnitin. (2023). *Turnitin services privacy policy.* https://help.turnitin.com/Privacy_and_Security/Privacy_and_Security.htm?Highlight=privacy%20policy

   Turnitin. (n.d.). *Accessibility.* https://www.turnitin.com/accessibility

   VoiceThread. (2023). *Privacy notice.* https://voicethread.com/privacy/

   VoiceThread. (n.d.). *Every one of us works differently.* https://voicethread.com/about/features/accessibility

REFERENCES

Bollinger, D., & Martin, F. (2021). Critical design elements in online courses. *Distance Education, 24*(3), 352–372. https://doi.org/10.1080/01587919.2021.1956301

Garrison, D. R., Anderson, T., & Archer, W. (2000). Critical inquiry in a text-based environment: Computer conferencing in higher education. *The Internet and Higher Education, 2*(2–3), 87–105. https://doi.org/10.1016/S1096-7516(00)00016

Gupta, A., Singh, S., Aravindakshan, R., & Kakkar, R. (2022). Netiquette and ethics regarding digital education across institutions: A narrative review. *Journal of Clinical & Diagnostic Research, 16*(11), 1–5. https://doi-10.7860/JCDR/2022/56978.17150

Instructure. (2023). *How do I link to other Canvas pages in a course?* https://community.canvaslms.com/t5/Instructor-Guide/How-do-I-link-to-other-Canvas-pages-in-a-course/

Jordan, T. (2022, August 15). *The role of instructional designer.* Instructional Design Central. https://www.instructionaldesigncentral.com/post/the-role-of-instructional-designer

Kaspersky. (2023). *What is netiquette* [Video]. YouTube. https://www.youtube.com/watch?v=CWbtbycHZok

Kaspersky. (2024). *Preemptive safety: What is netiquette? 20 internet etiquette rules.* https://usa.kaspersky.com/resource-center/preemptive-safety/what-is-netiquette

Konstantinidis, A. (2022). Analysis of design elements in universal course shell templates of high-ranking universities. *Knowledge Management & E-Learning, 14*(3), 344–359. https://doi.org/10.34105/j.kmel

McMullan, T., Williams, D., Ortiz, Y., & Lollar, J. (2021). Is consistency possible? Course design and delivery to meet faculty and student needs. *Current Issues in Education, 23*(3), 1–22.

Mikolon, T. M., Murphy, B. N., & Justice, E. (2022). The online syllabus: A means of communication to enhance student success. *Distance Learning, 19*(4), 69–80.

Moodle. (2023). https://moodle.org

Pappas, C. (2021, June 4). *7 top technical difficulties in online training and tips to get rid of the glitches.* eLearning Industry. https://elearningindustry.com/top-technical-difficulties-in-online-training-tips-get-rid-glitches

Ralston-Berg, P., & Braatz, H. (2021). Online course design structure and interface. *New Directions Adult Continuing Education, 2021*(169), 15–33. https://doi.org/10.1002/ace.20411

Richardson, J. C., Ashby, I., Alshammari, A. N., Cheng, Z., Johnson, B. S., Krause, T. S., Lee, D., Randolph, A. E., & Wang, H. (2019). Faculty and instructional designers on building successful collaborative relationships. *Educational Technology Research & Development*, 67(4), 855–880. https://doi-org/10.1007/s11423-018-9636-4

Sakai LMS. (2023). https://www.sakailms.org

Seckman, C. (2018). Impact of interactive video communication versus text-based feedback on teaching, social, and cognitive presence in online learning communities. *Nurse Educator, 43*(1), 18–22. https://doi.org/10.1097/NNE.0000000000000448

Wengier, S. (2022). The start here module: Creating a first-day impression in an online language class. *Dimension,* 35–56.

Wright, A. C., Carley, C., Alarakyia-Jivani, R., & Nizamuddin, S. (2023). Features of high-quality online courses in higher education: A scoping review. *Online Learning, 27*(1), 46–70. https://doi.org/10.24059/olj.v27i1.3411

Credits

Fig. 4.3: Source: Penny Ralston-Berg and Heather Braatz, "Online Course Design Structure and Interface," New Directions for Adult and Continuing Education, vol. 2021, no. 169, p. 21, 2021.

Icon 4.1: Apple icon is Copyright © by Microsoft.

Fig. 4.5a: Laptop is Copyright © 2013 Pixabay/OpenClipart-Vectors.

Icon 4.2: Owl icon is Copyright © by Microsoft.

Icon 4.3: Copyright © by Microsoft.

Icon 4.4: Slate icon is Copyright © by Microsoft.

Icon 4.5: Pencil icon is Copyright © by Microsoft.

Icon 4.6: Computer icon is Copyright © by Microsoft.

CHAPTER 5

Technology Tools

Application for Online Teaching and Learning

"Technology will never replace great teachers, but technology in the hands of great teachers is transformational."

—GEORGE COURAS
(INNOVATIVE TEACHING, LEARNING, AND LEADERSHIP CONSULTANT)

TERMS TO KNOW

academic dishonesty: The opposite of academic integrity; includes plagiarism, falsifying information, cheating on tests, misrepresentation of work and/or self, contract cheating, recycling one's own academic work, and uploading course materials to an external site.

academic integrity: The act of upholding the values of honesty, responsibility, respect, fairness, trust, and courage in one's academic work and applying these values to coursework, scholarship, and research.

app: The short word for *application*. For this chapter, an app is a software product and a type of educational tool that is installed, downloaded, or available through the learning management system (LMS) to assist with online teaching–learning activities.

artificial intelligence (AI): A technology that enables computers and machines to simulate human intelligence and problem-solving capabilities.

contract cheating: When a student pays for or downloads external material and presents it as their own academic work.

educational technology tool: Any digital resource that enhances or assists with the teaching–learning process. Technology tools include apps, platforms, and software specific for education.

Chapter Overview and Objectives

This chapter provides information about common educational technology tools used in the online teaching–learning environment. Learners identify categories of technology tools and apps and apply them to online teaching–learning situations. Examples of technology tools and apps are software products for use in the learning management system (LMS), student tools and apps for assignments and for assistance with learning disabilities, virtual communication and meeting tools, online collaboration and project-creation tools, and assessment and evaluation tools. The chapter presents the use of plagiarism tools in conjunction with a discussion about academic dishonesty and concludes with introductory information about the use of artificial intelligence (AI) in online education.

In this chapter, the learner will:

1. Identify categories of educational technology tools and apps.
2. Utilize a rubric to assess the strengths and weaknesses of educational technology tools.
3. Apply appropriate technology tools and apps for online teaching–learning scenarios.
4. Examine the use of and indications for testing and antiplagiarism software in the online teaching–learning environment.
5. Formulate a plan to encourage academic honesty in the online classroom.
6. Contribute to the discussion about the use of AI technology in academia.

Educational Technology Tools and Apps

Nurse faculty use various teaching strategies supported by educational technology, which comprises any digital resource that enhances or assists with the teaching-learning process. Technology tools include applications (apps), platforms, and software specific for education. The market for educational technology tools is expanding and changing. A quick internet search on "educational technology" reveals hundreds of examples of apps and tools categorized for appropriate use in the online teaching-learning environment.

Tools and apps for learning have numerous benefits for both the faculty and the online learner in the virtual setting. In addition to online course delivery formatting, the faculty can use educational technology to support innovative teaching actions for assignments, assessments, activities, content presentation, and testing. In addition, educational technology benefits students with hearing, speech, and reading disabilities (see apps that were reviewed in Chapter 4). The advantages of educational apps and tools for online students range from self-assessment of learning to online community building. Khalid et al. (2024) highlight the use of interactive educational technology in nursing curricula, which has cognitive advantages for students and the added benefits of self-regulation, self-efficacy, and motivation. Additional examples of benefits of educational technology are provided in Box 5.1.

Application of Tools and Apps for Online Teaching-Learning

Online teaching-learning tools and apps can be grouped into several categories. There are general tools for the online classroom for assignments and activities. Other apps and tools are grouped according to use for accessibility, communication, online collaboration, project creation, assessment and evaluation, plagiarism, and online testing. Teaching-learning tools and apps are commonly available through learning management systems (LMSs); through university, program, or library purchase agreements; and/or offered for trial use by specific technology companies. Many educational technology companies charge a fee, either monthly or annually; others charge per project; and some offer a free version of their app or tool. Apps are abundant. For example, Microsoft 365 Education has a drop-down menu of writing app "add-ins" located at the top right corner of the Microsoft Word document ribbon. Universities may purchase apps and tools for online programs and embed them in the LMS for faculty and student use. For example, a school can insert a video application into every course that uses the LMS. Faculty may want to use apps and tools that are not embedded and can download an app or tool for an individual course, if needed. Table 5.1 provides examples of tools and apps appropriate for online teaching and learning. For a directory of educational tools and apps, check out the link in the Chapter Resources at the end of the chapter.

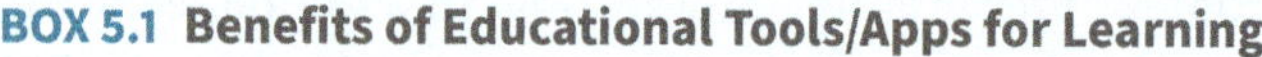

BOX 5.1 Benefits of Educational Tools/Apps for Learning

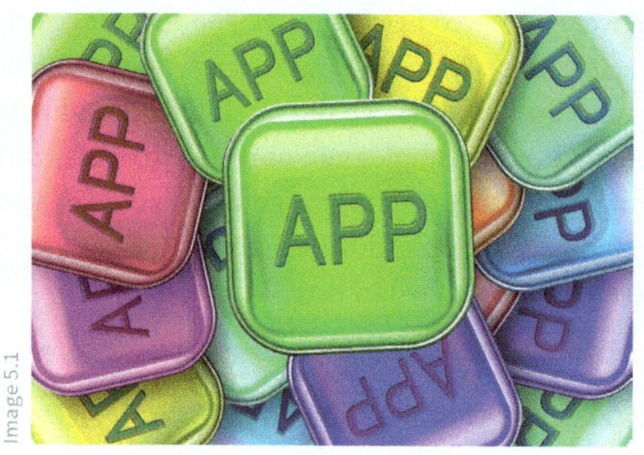

Image 5.1

- Promote online engagement.
- Encourage collaboration.
- Foster a sense of community.
- Enhance ability to gather information.
- Enhance ability to organize information.
- Augment student presentations.
- Facilitate communication.
- Facilitate meetings.
- Promote learning of new digital skills.
- Promote self-assessment (e.g., grammar, spelling).

TABLE 5.1 Sample Apps for Online Learning

App/Tool Category	App/Tool Examples	Indications	More information and app/ tool comparisons
General tools for assignments and activities/	Khan Academy: https://www.khanacademy.org Evernote: https://evernote.com/ Classpoint games and interactive exercises: https://www.classpoint.io/gamification	Assignments Organization and notetaking Presentations and integration of assignments	https://www.classpoint.io/blog/edtech-tools-for-higher-education
Accessibility apps and tools	CBoardacc: https://www.cboard.io/about/ Asoft: https://www.a-soft.nl/ Abbyy Textgraber: https://pdf.abbyy.com/products/mobile/text-grabber/en/	Transcription services Captioning services Speech recognition services Text-to-speech screen reader Refreshable Braille readers Assisted reading applications Screen magnifiers	https://www.rev.com/blog/speech-to-text-accessibility/7-web-accessibility-resources-every-college-with-distance-learning-needs

(Continued)

TABLE 5.1 (Continued)

App/Tool Category	App/Tool Examples	Indications	More information and app/tool comparisons
Communication apps	MS Teams: https://www.microsoft.com/en-us/microsoft-teams/group-chat-software Zoom: https://zoom.us Slack: https://slack.com	Virtual meetings: group or one on one Voice and video calling	https://connecteam.com/best-team-communication-apps/
Online / collaboration tools	Padlet: https://padlet.com Slack: https://slack.com	Group work Paired assignments Communication and collaboration	https://clickup.com/blog/collaboration-tools-students/
Project-creation tools	Prezi: https://prezi.com PowerPoint: https://www.microsoft.com/en-us/microsoft-365/powerpoint Kaltura Capture (a desktop recorder that is embedded in the course): https://knowledge.kaltura.com/help/kaltura-capture-overview iMovie: https://imovie-app.com YouTube Creators: https://www.youtube.com/creators/	Online classroom presentations Recording audio and or video	https://www.simplilearn.com/project-management-apps-article

TABLE 5.1 (Continued)

App/Tool Category	App/Tool Examples	Indications	More information and app/tool comparisons
Assessment and evaluation tools and apps	Examsoft: https://examsoft.com/	Test/quiz construction Data collection and test construction	https://www.ispring-solutions.com/blog/8-ways-to-assess-online-student-learning https://www.capterra.com/exam-software/
Plagiarism and academic integrity tools	Respondus Lockdown Browser: https://web.respondus.com/he/lockdownbrowser/ Turnitin: https://www.turnitin.com/products/similarity/ Honorlock: https://honorlock.com/faculty/	Secure online exams Check similarity against published material Online proctoring	https://www.ispring-solutions.com/blog/free-online-plagiarism-checkers-for-teachers-and-educators

Not all apps are appropriate for online learning in higher education. Faculty should assess each educational app and tool for usability and applicability to the course content. Anstey and Watson (2018) created a rubric to assess educational technology apps and tools across categories such as functionality, accessibility, technology, mobile design, social presence, privacy, teacher presence, and cognitive presence. The chosen app is compared to the criteria in each category of the rubric to determine strengths and weaknesses (Anstey & Watson, 2018). See the Chapter Resources for a link to the rubric.

Course/Content Application

After assessing the apps for strengths and weaknesses, faculty can decide which apps and tools are appropriate for course assignments, activities, and assessments. The following examples demonstrate how faculty can incorporate multiple apps and tools for specific assignments.

Example 1

An asynchronous online nursing leadership course uses a paired-student assignment. Students select a leadership book to read and pair up to present the book using leadership concepts that apply to the healthcare setting. Appropriate apps for the students to use for meetings and communication to plan the book presentation include Zoom or MS Teams. To prepare the presentation, students could use Slack or Padlet to collaborate; the apps allow each student to work asynchronously on the book presentation. In addition, students could collaborate asynchronously on the presentation using MS 365 in a shared virtual drive. PowerPoint and Prezi are examples of tools used to create and present the final assignment; either would be appropriate for this activity. Students can use an app such as Kaltura Capture to record the presentation. The websites for the example tools are provided in the Table 5.1.

Example 2

An online asynchronous population health nursing course assignment requires students to take a picture or make a short 2-minute video that represents an aspect of environmental impact on human health. Students meet one-on-one with faculty to present a 10-minute oral discussion of the negative influence of this representation of the environment from a human health or population health perspective. In addition, the student discusses ideas for public policy and planning to prevent future harm to population health. Examples of appropriate apps for the students to use for creating videos are iMovie, Kaltura, and YouTube Creators. The student can upload the video or picture to their computer. Faculty can use Zoom for the students to present the issues along with the video or picture presentation. Students can show their video or picture during the presentation using the Zoom share screen feature or through the file upload feature.

Faculty Apps

Faculty may choose to build their own app for an assignment, course content, or for learning assistance. A variety of no-code app builders specifically designed for education are available. *No code* means that the app can be created or built without the use of computer language. No-code app builders use templates so that faculty can drag and drop content and update information as needed in the app. Jotform is an example of a free no-code app builder with templates appropriate for educational levels K through college for use in the online classroom (https://www.jotform.com/app-templates/category/education-app-templates). Faculty-created apps should be held to the same standards as proprietary apps. Faculty can use the Rubric for eLearning Tool (Anstey & Watson, 2018) to determine the strengths and weaknesses of any educational app they develop. Furthermore, every app that is used in the online environment should have an accessibility and a privacy statement posted on the LMS site. The best place for these statements is in the "Start Here" area of the course or module 0 (see Chapter 4).

Academic Dishonesty Issues and Testing and Plagiarism Software

Academic integrity is upholding the six values of honesty, responsibility, respect, fairness, trust, and courage (International Center for Academic Integrity [ICAI], 2021) in one's academic work, which applies to coursework, scholarship, and research. In other words, all students, including those in the online environment, are expected to do their own coursework and assignments, take their own tests, represent their own ideas, provide references for others' work, and not share course materials on external websites. Academic dishonesty violates academic integrity through actions such as plagiarism, falsifying information, cheating on tests, misrepresentation of work and or self, contract cheating, reusing one's own academic work, and uploading course materials to an external site. For more information about academic integrity, review the document *The Fundamental Values of Academic Integrity* (see Chapter Resources). The document examines the six values and presents strategies to promote academic integrity in the academic environment.

SHOW WHAT YOU KNOW ASSIGNMENT

Directions: Continue to construct your course map. Review resources at the links in Table 5.1 for app ideas and add appropriate apps and tools in the green space that align with Unit 1/Module 1 on the map. Share your ideas with your peers.

Name of course: Translation and Utilization of Evidence for Nursing Practice		
Units	**Unit 1**	**Unit 2**
Unit title//topic		
End-of-program outcome(s) (EPO)		
Course objective(s) (CO)		
Unit objective(s) (UO)		

Assignment/activity (List one or more activities for each week or unit, as appropriate. Label the unit objective that aligns with the assignment/activity.)	
Assessment/evaluation (List one or more assessments for each week or unit, as appropriate. Label with the unit objective that aligns with the assessment activity.)	
High-impact practice	
Principles of universal design	
Inclusive design	
Online tools/apps	Review resources at the links in Table 5.1 and add apps here.

Studies by Dr. Donald McCabe over the past three decades highlight the pervasiveness of academic dishonesty in the higher education environment, with 60 percent of students in higher education acknowledging engaging in some type of cheating (ICAI, 2024). Rettinger et al. (2022) updated McCabe's study and found that 32 percent of college students admitted to cheating on an exam, 25 percent used unapproved e-resources for coursework and assignments, 28 percent collaborated on assignments that required individual work, and 18 percent reported plagiarizing other's work (ICAI, 2024; Rettinger, 2022). Academic dishonesty occurs in nursing education (Bultas et al., 2017; McClung & Gaberson, 2021) and in both the traditional classroom and the online learning environment, with similar actions such as plagiarism, falsifying information, cheating on tests, misrepresentation of work and self, and contract cheating (Monahan & Shah, 2023; Surahman & Wang, 2022). In a study of 319 online undergraduate health students, 82 percent admitted to some form of academic dishonesty in the year previous and 77 percent observed the same behaviors in peers (Hasri et al., 2022). Online students engage in academic dishonesty for a variety of reasons, some of which are listed in Box 5.2.

BOX 5.2 Reasons Online Students Engage in Academic Dishonesty

Amigud and Lancaster (2019):

- Lack of preparedness
- Lack of social support
- Family and work responsibility
- Lack of self-discipline
- Inability to follow through

Valizadeh (2022):

- Lack of knowledge
- Want better grades
- Technical issues
- Lack of or insufficient proctoring
- Stress about the test

Jenkins et al. (2023):

- Hard classes
- Not prepared
- Busy with work
- COVID-19
- Pressure
- Stress
- No time

Adzima (2020):

- Anonymity in online learning
- Easy to cheat online
- Lax teaching–learning setting
- Lack of knowledge about plagiarism
- Relaxed attitude toward contract cheating
- Difficult course or instructor

Contract Cheating and Antiplagiarism Tools

Online students may engage in contract cheating, which is the action of outsourcing assignments, tests, and other academic work to someone else, usually for a price (Amigud & Lancaster, 2019; Clarke & Lancaster, 2006). Online contract cheating companies provide essays, presentations, and assignments for students. These companies generate billions of dollars in revenue (Velliaris, 2020). A quick internet search of "homework help," "essay help," and "exam help" reveals a plethora of company websites advertising these services. The contract cheating companies use social media and other legitimate-looking advertisements and websites to entice students to use their services (Rowland et al., 2018) and then charge students for services; in some cases, the companies engage in blackmail for additional money (Palmer, 2024; Velliaris, 2020; Yorke et al., 2022). It is a challenge for faculty to determine when students submit documents from these companies because the author source is removed from the document properties and the assignments are not flagged by antiplagiarism software.

Online educational honesty tools are placed in courses and in the LMS to detect and discourage academic dishonesty. Antiplagiarism tools, testing software, and lockdown browsers are all designed to hinder academic dishonesty. The functions of the different tools are to check similarity against published materials, provide online proctoring, and secure online exams, respectively. Even with the presence of the tools in online courses, students develop workarounds. Jenkins et al. (2023) reported that of the 85 percent of students who stated that faculty used software to prevent academic dishonesty, 16 percent of these students attempted to work around the software. At one university, an instructional designer in collaboration with a faculty teaching a math course posed as a student and contracted with a cheating company to take an online exam; the contract cheating company bypassed the proctoring software and took the online math exam for the "student" behind the scenes while the proctoring video portrayed the "student" taking the computerized exam, thus demonstrating that cheating companies can circumvent testing software (Palmer, 2024).

Despite faculty good intentions, students find ways to cheat, either alone or with the assistance of contract cheating companies. No academic honesty tool is foolproof, and therefore should be considered as the last line of defense. Academic dishonesty diminishes the academic experience; therefore, faculty should focus on designing an online course where students feel less compelled to cheat. Good online pedagogy should be directed toward the appropriate presentation of the content, less high-stakes assessments, more interaction between faculty and students, and student opportunities to demonstrate knowledge in ways other than essays or exams. Faculty can place the university honor code/academic integrity statement in the syllabus and other prominent places in the online course. Also, faculty can write an honesty statement specific for their online course, discuss the statement expectations, and require the students to read and sign the statement. Additional strategies for decreasing academic dishonesty are found in the *Teacher Tidbits.*

TEACHER TIDBITS TO DECREASE ACADEMIC DISHONESTY IN ONLINE COURSES

- Discuss academic integrity and remind students to:
  - Express independent ideas.
  - Cite information from all sources.
  - Ensure that exams and assignments are one's own work.
- Review the American Nurses Association (ANA) code of ethics in the course (ANA, 2015).
- Be flexible with due dates.
- Develop students' writing skills.
  - Discuss paraphrasing.
  - Allow for peer review.
  - Provide a supportive environment.
  - Encourage multiple drafts and provide feedback.
- Support students' well-being.
- Provide rubrics that align with material and course outcomes.
- Use interactive assignments.

- Maintain faculty presence.
- Encourage interaction between faculty and students.
- Provide reminders about academic integrity.
- Consider alternatives to exams.
- Use a variety of assignments and assessments.
- Use scaffolding assignments.
- Change assignments each semester.
- Change discussion board questions frequently.
- Address dishonesty immediately.

Adapted from: McGee, P. (2013). Supporting academic honesty in online courses. *Journal of Educators Online*, *10*(1), 1–31. https://doi-org/10.9743/JEO.2013.1.6; Smith, K., Grugan, A., Ott, M. N., Borton, R., & Reed, S. (2023). Strategies to promote academic integrity for graduate nursing students in an online learning environment. *Distance Learning*, *20*(1), 19–23. https://www.infoagepub.com/products/distance-learning-vol-20-1; Tatum, H., & Schwartz, B. M. (2017). Honor codes: Evidence based strategies for improving academic integrity. *Theory Into Practice*, *56*(2), 129–135. https://doi-org/10.1080/00405841.2017.1308175

Artificial Intelligence and Academic Dishonesty

Artificial intelligence (AI) is a technology that enables computers and machines to simulate human intelligence and problem-solving capabilities (IBM, n.d.). There are four types of AI: type 1 relative machine AI, type 2 limited-memory AI, type 3 theory of mind AI, and type 4 self-aware AI (IBM, 2023). As of spring 2024, type 3 and 4 are currently under development and are discussed in Chapter 10. Type 1, which is machine AI, uses algorithms to automatically learn about and recognize patterns from data; which exponentially allows AI to make better choices and decisions. A more developed type 1 AI is deep learning, where machines function similarly to neural pathways in the brain to analyze data; these machines incorporate brainlike logic to learn more intricate patterns to make independent decisions and predictions without human involvement (Columbia Engineering, 2024). Companies have developed type 2 AI systems for generating written information, images, and videos, among other uses. Select examples of type 2 AI applicable to student and faculty work are ChatGPT (https://chat.openai.com), Claude AI (https://claude.ai./login), and Bing Chat (https://bing.com), which have the specific task of text-based chat. Since spring 2023, the use of AI in higher education has been a hot topic. The challenges around AI are primarily acceptance of its application in the academic environment; specifically, that students will use chat AI to create papers and complete assignments. Topics to consider are how much students will use AI, and how much use is acceptable? According to the *Inside Higher Ed* 2024 Annual Provost survey, only 1 in 5 universities or colleges have an official policy about the use of AI in research or teaching (Quinn, 2024). Conversation in the literature for faculty encompasses the balance between promoting AI skill development for students and issues around originality and writing (Enis, 2023; Walczak & Cellary, 2023). At present, plagiarism tools have AI detection capabilities, but vary in their level of accuracy (Walters, 2023), so the advice to faculty is not to rely solely on the data from the plagiarism tool.

Students use AI more readily than faculty. A fall 2023 study of 1,600 students and 1,000 faculty in postsecondary settings found that almost 50 percent of students surveyed use generative AI, compared to 22 percent of faculty; in addition, 33 percent of students would be somewhat likely, 23 percent likely, and 19 percent extremely likely to use AI in their academic work even if faculty prohibited its use (Bharadwaj et al., 2023). The forecast is that AI will become more robust as more information is consumed by AI technology (IBM, 2023). Faculty can be forward-thinking and develop recommendations for AI use in the online classroom. Select strategies are to (1) create guidelines for AI use, (2) review ethics of using AI (e.g., discuss appropriate use for incorporation of AI into one's own work, such as acceptable use for assignments), and (3) discuss the limitations of AI, such as bias and inaccuracies (Mowreader, 2024). Faculty are urged to be well informed about the use and future of AI in the online higher education learning environment. In the interim, faculty are encouraged to use current information to develop activities and assignments using AI that will teach students new skills, teach critical-thinking actions, and promote discernment pertaining to AI. See Box 5.3 for an example of an appropriate AI assignment. The example incorporates the faculty strategies discussed, including directions for use of AI information.

BOX 5.3 AI Assignment Example

Assignment Background: As part of a leader-challenge oral presentation, students are tasked with providing recommendations to manage a current or anticipated system problem or challenge within a healthcare organization. These recommendations are to be supported with concepts from current research. Recent developments in AI have brought about new and powerful ways to research a topic. Although fast and thorough, these new tools have drawbacks and flaws that may not be readily apparent. Part of this assignment will be to see how useful new AI tools can be and how they compare to more traditional research methods you may be used to.

What tool should I use?

The AI tool you'll be using for this course is Elicit (https://elicit.com). Give yourself time to familiarize yourself with this tool on the site.

On the main page of Elicit, you can ask a research question or topic question in natural language. Elicit will then attempt to understand the meaning of your question and find articles related to it.

How do I use Elicit?

After asking Elicit a question, you can review the papers/articles it provides and the abstract summary. Try asking direct and simple questions first, then move to more complex questions and determine the difference in Elicit's quality of articles.

You can filter Elicit's results by article date, keywords, whether it has a readable PDF (important if you do not have access to the article otherwise!), and even by study type!

You can also add more information than just the summary. On the left side, you will see "Add information about all papers" and can add in other information, such as a more detailed abstract summary, limitations, outcomes measured, number of participants, methodology, and more. Just click in the "Search for paper information" search box to find more options.

What do I submit?

Submit a one-page summary of the experience using Elicit to find your topic for your leadership challenge. Answer the following questions in your summary:

- What questions did you ask Elicit to find articles on your topic? Include both the simple and complex questions that you used to obtain your results. The results are the articles on your topic.
- What advantages did you find using Elicit for researching your topic? What disadvantages?
- What errors did you find in Elicit's findings (e.g., incorrect or omitted authors, incorrect or incomplete abstract summaries, etc.)?
    - How did you locate these errors? What was your process for determining if the articles were strong evidence to support your oral presentation?
- What did you look for in Elicit's results to determine if a paper was useful enough to research further? (Abstract, paper title, participant number, etc.)
- Will you use the information in your oral presentation? Why or why not?
- Submit this summary along with the list of references that you will use in your oral presentation one day before your scheduled presentation.

Conclusion

Educational apps and tools can enhance learning when employed appropriately. The use of educational technology tools for online teaching-learning requires knowledge about their indications and applications for use. Faculty can review apps and tools appropriate for the online environment and finalize decisions for use with a rubric to assess the strengths and weaknesses of each technology. Tools to discourage plagiarism and other forms of academic dishonesty should be used judiciously due to student workarounds and the use of contract cheating companies; however, faculty can use online classroom strategies to deter academic dishonesty. The discussion about the use of AI in higher education is evolving, so faculty are encouraged to stay informed as the technology develops.

TAKE 5

List five take-away points from Chapter 5.

What did you learn?

1.
2.
3.
4.
5.

What additional information do you need to understand the concepts? See the Chapter Resources for additional material.

CHAPTER ACTIVITIES

1. Use the websites and resources provided in the chapter or browse the internet to choose an appropriate technology tool or tools for a specific online teaching and learning scenario such as an assignment, test, quiz, or online course activity.
2. Complete the "Show What You Assignment" and add appropriate apps and tools to the evolving course map.
3. Create an academic honesty statement for a syllabus for a course that you are currently enrolled in or for one that you plan to teach in the future.
4. Develop an online assignment that incorporates a suitable AI tool.
5. **Caring on Sharing.** In your journal, provide an update on the self-care activity.

CHAPTER RESOURCES

1. Directory of education tools from eLearning Industry: https://elearningindustry.com/directory/software-categories/elearning-authoring-tools

2. *Rubric for eLearning tool evaluation* by Anstey and Watson: https://teaching.uwo.ca/pdf/elearning/Rubric-for-eLearning-Tool-Evaluation.pdf
3. *The fundamental values of academic integrity* (3rd ed): https://academicintegrity.org/images/pdfs/20019_ICAI-Fundamental-Values_R12.pdf
4. GenAI in higher education: Fall 2023 update time for class study: Bharadwaj, P., Shaw, C., NeJame, L., Martin, S., Janson, N., & Fox, K. (2023, June). *Time for Class - 2023.* Tyton Partners. https://tytonpartners.com/time-for-class-2023-bridging-student-and-faculty-perspectives-on-digital-learning/

REFERENCES

Abbyy. (2022). *Text grabber.* Abbyy. https://pdf.abbyy.com/products/mobile/text-grabber/en/

Adzima, K. (2020). Examining online cheating in higher education using traditional classroom cheating as a guide. *Electronic Journal of E-Learning, 18*(6), 476–493. https://doi-/10.34190/JEL.18.6.002

American Nurses Association. (2015). *ANA code of ethics with interpretive statements.* https://www.nursingworld.org/practice-policy/nursing-excellence/ethics/code-of-ethics-for-nurses/

Amigud, A., & Lancaster, T. (2019). 246 reasons to cheat: An analysis of students' reasons for seeking to outsource academic work. *Computers & Education, 134*, 98–107. https://doi-/10.1016/j.compedu.2019.01.017

Anstey, L., & Watson., G. (2018). A rubric for evaluating e-learning tools in higher education. *Educause Review.* https://er.educause.edu/articles/2018/9/a-rubric-for-evaluating-e-learning-tools-in-higher-education

Bharadwaj, P., Shaw, C., NeJame, L., Martin, S., Janson, N., & Fox, K. (2023, June). *Time for Class - 2023.* Tyton Partners. https://tytonpartners.com/time-for-class-2023-bridging-student-and-faculty-perspectives-on-digital-learning/

Bultas, M. W., Schmuke, A. D., Davis, R. L., & Palmer, J. L. (2017). Crossing the "line": College students and academic integrity in nursing. *Nurse Education Today, 56*, 57–62. https://doi.org/ 10.1016/j.nedt.2017.06.012

Clarke, R., & Lancaster, T. (2006). Eliminating the successor to plagiarism? Identifying the usage of contract cheating sites. *Proceedings of 2nd International Plagiarism Conference, June 19–21.* Northumbria Learning Press.

Clickup. (2024). *10 best online collaboration tools for students in 2024.* Clickup Engineering Team. https://clickup.com/blog/collaboration-tools-students/

Columbia Engineering. (2024). *Artificial intelligence (AI) vs. machine learning.* https://ai.engineering.columbia.edu/ai-vs-machine-learning/

Couras, C. (2024). *Learner speaker author.* https://georgecouros.ca/blog/about-me/

eLearning Industry. (2024). *Directory: eLearning authoring tools.* https://elearningindustry.com/directory/software-categories/elearning-authoring-tools

Enis, M. (2023, May 1). Perspectives on AI in higher ed. *Library Journal, 148*(5).

Hasri, A., Supar, R., Dizyana, N., Azman, N., Sharip, H., & Yamin, L. S. M. (2022). Students' attitudes and behavior towards academic dishonesty during online learning. *Proceedings, 82,* 36. https://doi.org/10.3390/proceedings2022082036

IBM. (n.d.) *What is artificial intelligence (AI)?* https://www.ibm.com/topics/artificial-intelligence

IBM. (2023). *Understanding the different types of artificial intelligence.* https://www.ibm.com/blog/understanding-the-different-types-of-artificial-intelligence/

International Center for Academic Integrity. (2021). *The fundamental values of academic integrity.* (3rd ed). https://academicintegrity.org/images/pdfs/20019_ICAI-Fundamental-Values_R12.pdf

International Center for Academic Integrity. (2024). *Facts and statistics.* https://academicintegrity.org/esources/facts-and-statistics

Jenkins, B. D., Golding, J. M., Le Grand, A. M., Levi, M. M., & Pals, A. M. (2023). When opportunity knocks: College students' cheating amid the COVID-19 pandemic. *Teaching of Psychology, 50*(4), 407–419. https://doi-org/10.1177/00986283211059067

Jotform App Builder. (2024). *Education app templates.* https://www.jotform.com/app-templates/category/education-app-templates

Khalid, N., Zapparrata, N., & Cusatis Phillips, B. (2024). Theoretical underpinnings of technology-based interactive instruction. *Teaching and Learning in Nursing, 19*(1), e145–e149. https://doi.org/10.1016/j.teln.2023.10.004

McClung, E. L., & Gaberson, K. B. (2021). Academic dishonesty among nursing students: A contemporary view. *Nurse Educator, 46*(2), 111–115. https://doi10.1097/NNE.0000000000000863

McGee, P. (2013). Supporting academic honesty in online courses. *Journal of Educators Online, 10*(1), 1–31. https://doi-org/10.9743/JEO.2013.1.6

Monahan, M., & Shah, A. (2023). Academic dishonesty: An exploratory study of traditional versus non-traditional students. *Research in Higher Education Journal, 43.* Retrieved from https://eric.ed.gov/?id=EJ1382877

Mowreader, A. (2024, February 6). Teaching tip: Navigating AI in the classroom. *Insider Higher Ed.* https://www.insidehighered.com/news/student-success/academic-life/2024/02/06/how-college-professors-are-using-generative-ai-teach

Palmer, K. (2024, March 28). Sting operation fools a proctoring service—and results in blackmail attempt. *Inside Higher Ed.* https://www.insidehighered.com/news/students/academics/2024/03/28/sting-operation-fools-proctoring-service-blackmail-attempted#

Quinn, R. (2024, April, 16). Annual provosts' survey shows need for AI policies, worries over campus speech. *Inside Higher Ed.* https://www.insidehighered.com/news/tech-innovation/artificial-intelligence/2024/04/16/provosts-survey-shows-need-ai-policies?utm_source=Inside+Higher+Ed

Rettinger, D., & Bertram Gallant, T. (2022). Thirty years of active academic integrity research and engagement: What have we learned? *Journal of College & Character, 23*(1), 92–95. https://doi.org/10.1080/2194587X.2021.2017976

Rowland, S., Slade, C., Wong, K.-S., & Whiting, B. (2018). "Just turn to us": The persuasive features of contract cheating websites. *Assessment & Evaluation in Higher Education, 43*(4), 652–665. https://doi- org/10.1080/02602938.2017.1391948

Simplilearn. (2023). *20+ most widely used project management apps compared.* https://www.simplilearn.com/project-management-apps-article

Smith, K., Grugan, A., Ott, M. N., Borton, R., & Reed, S. (2023). Strategies to promote academic integrity for graduate nursing students in an online learning environment. *Distance Learning, 20*(1), 19–23. https://www.infoagepub.com/products/distance-learning-vol-20-1

Surahman, E., & Wang, T. H. (2022). Academic dishonesty and trustworthy assessment in online learning: A systematic literature review. *Journal of Computer Assisted Learning, 38,*1535–1553. https://doi.org/10.1111/jcal.12708

Tatum, H., & Schwartz, B. M. (2017). Honor codes: Evidence based strategies for improving academic integrity. *Theory Into Practice, 56*(2), 129–135. https://doi-org/10.1080/00405841.2017.1308175

Taylor, R. (2020). *7 web accessibility resources every college with distance learning needs.* Rev. https://www.rev.com/blog/speech-to-text-accessibility/7-web-accessibility-resources-every-college-with-distance-learning-needs

Valizadeh, M. (2022). Cheating in online learning programs: Learners' perceptions and solutions. *Turkish Online Journal of Distance Education (TOJDE), 23*(1), 195–209. https://doi-/10.17718/tojde.1050394

Velliaris, D. (2020). *Contract cheating: A billion dollar industry.* [Newsroom]. IGI Global. https://www.igi-global.com/newsroom/archive/contract-cheating-billion-dollar-industry/4617/

Walczak, K., & Cellary, W. (2023). Challenges for higher education in the era of widespread access to generative AI. *Economics & Business Review, 9*(2), 71–100. https://doi-.org/10.18559/ebr.2023.2.743

Walters, W. (2023). The effectiveness of software designed to detect ai-generated writing: A comparison of 16 AI text detectors. *Open Information Science, 7.* https://doi.org/10.1515/opis-2022-0158

Yankovsky, D. (2024). *The 10 best team communication apps for 2024.* Connecteam. https://connecteam.com/best-team-communication-apps/

Yorke, J., Sefcik, L., & Veeran-Colton, T. (2022). Contract cheating and blackmail: A risky business? *Studies in Higher Education, 47*(1), 53–66. https://doi-/10.1080/03075079.2020.1730313

Credits

PART II

Online Nursing Education as Art

Virtual Teaching, Learning, and Caring

CHAPTER 6

Caring, Communication, and Social Presence in Online Nursing Education

"Caring is the intentional attention to making a connection with a student."

—ONLINE GRADUATE NURSING STUDENT

TERMS TO KNOW

instructor/faculty immediacy: Verbal and nonverbal actions that may close the gap of perceived distance by the students. Examples of immediacy behaviors are eye contact, vocal intonation and variation, facial expressions, relaxed body posture, and gestures that personalize interactions in the learning environment. Faculty strategies such as use of video meetings, video and audio course content materials, phone calls, announcements, positive emails, and presenting as authentic self are all opportunities for faculty immediacy in the virtual educational setting.

online communication: Construction of online messages that include a sender and a receiver; a feedback loop or reaction to the message completes the cycle. Online communication takes many forms, such as text, email messages, and video and audio messages, and influences student-to-faculty interactions, student-to-student interactions, and student-to-course interactions.

online social presence: A form of faculty/instructor immediacy; the process of exhibiting oneself as human in the online environment through the display of emotions and social actions. Use of emotion, addressing students by their preferred name, and using thoughtful, caring, positive, and authentic words are examples of social presence applicable to the online teaching–learning environment.

Chapter Overview and Objectives

This chapter reviews principles for teaching online guided by select caring theories and introduces the learner to caring and social presence in online education from both the student and faculty perspectives. Research that supports caring actions for student success in online learning environments is explored. Activities that demonstrate faculty caring actions and social presence online that demonstrate empathetic and authentic communication, supportive guidance, timely and respectful feedback, and other behaviors are presented. Learners explore how to incorporate caring actions into a course map, convey caring in communication, enhance their faculty presence, demonstrate immediacy in the online teaching–learning setting, and troubleshoot miscommunication and technology issues that may interfere with online caring practices.

In this chapter, the learner will:

1. Identify the influence of caring theories and models in online teaching–learning environments.
2. Explain research findings that support online faculty caring and presence for student success.
3. Compare and contrast activities that support faculty caring actions in the online learning environment.
4. Demonstrate examples of faculty social presence and faculty immediacy in the online environment.
5. Troubleshoot technology and miscommunication issues that may interfere with online faculty caring actions.

Caring Theory and Online Education in Nursing

The notion of caring and the act of "being present" are characteristic of the nursing profession and are likely concepts found in nursing education curricula. These concepts transcend to the classroom; faculty demonstrate caring for students, and students display compassion for each other. Hayne et al. (2020) present a caring model for nursing education and propose that caring "permeates every aspect of the organization ... [and] is characterized by a relationship of trust among individuals, feelings of being valued, and having an ability to care among the faculty, and with students' perceptions that others care about them" (p. 10). In the virtual environment, faculty caring and online presence are challenged by lack of face-to-face interactions with students; technological difficulties; and, for some programs, the asynchronous nature of online course delivery. Select caring theories/frameworks appropriate to online learning are discussed here.

Human caring theories, originally developed for nursing practice and traditional face-to-face learning, can be directly applied to online teaching and learning environments. *Caring* is defined as "feeling or showing concern for or kindness to others" (Merriam-Webster, 2024, para. 1). However, in nursing theory circles, caring is described as much more, for example, as a human way of being or living (Roach, 2001). Caring is fundamental to the practice of the art of nursing; nurses employ caring as central in attending to the health needs of patients, families, and communities. Caring occurs anywhere; in nursing education, it is linked to student and faculty satisfaction and student success. Nurse educators demonstrate caring about students, which extends to the online teaching-learning environment and the implementation of the nursing education curriculum. Presented here are examples of how select caring theories and models apply to the online teaching-learning setting; the theories guide the work of nurse educators in planning and implementing online teaching strategies while at the same time demonstrating caring and presence.

The theory of human caring (Watson, 1985) is associated with 10 caritas processes, which are practices for nurses in caring for self and others. The caritas processes have broad application beyond practice, including education (Watson, 1997). Sitzman and Watson (2017) extended the caritas process into the virtual or cyber world and provide actions for the work, termed as *cybercaring*, demonstrated in Table 6.1.

Boykin and Schoenhofer's nursing as caring model (2001) posits that the nurse views and experiences self and others as living and growing in caring. The six assumptions foundational to nursing as caring are:

1. Persons are caring by virtue of their humanness.
2. Persons are whole or complete in the moment.
3. Persons live caring moment to moment.
4. Personhood is the process of living grounded in caring.
5. Personhood is enhanced through participating in nurturing relationships with caring others.
6. Nursing is both a discipline and profession. (p. 11)

In the nursing as caring model by Boykin & Schoenhofer (2001), nurse educators and administrators and nursing students are described as being in a dance of a caring circle. Using the model for nursing education means that the curriculum is grounded in caring principles. Faculty create a supportive learning environment that demonstrates appreciation for individual differences in caring actions and in personal and professional growth; in addition, faculty encourage caring through acceptance, risk-taking, sharing nursing stories, and self-reflection.

Sister Simone Roach (1992) emphasizes that caring is central to nursing, as demonstrated by five professional attributes known as the five Cs of caring: competence, confidence, conscience, compassion, and commitment. Roach writes that with these five attributes "specific manifestations of caring are actualized" (p. 67). The five attributes encompass the art and science of nursing and are applicable to the online educational setting.

Care, specifically culturally congruent care, is a major construct of Madeline Leininger's theory of culture care diversity and universality (Leininger, 1991; Leininger & McFarland, 2005). Leininger's theory maintains that caring assists or supports "individuals or groups to improve a human condition" (Leininger, 1991, p. 46), and that culturally congruent care is necessary for health and healing. The theory has been applied to a variety of settings, including nursing education, and supports care through three culture care decision and action modes; these decision action modes are Leininger's three theoretical modes of care for developing therapeutic relationships: (1) preservation and maintenance, (2) accommodation and negotiation, and (3) repatterning and restructuring (Leininger, 1991; McFarland & Wehbe-Alamah, 2018). The theory posits that nurse educators can support care and be present for students in the online environment; the online care is based on the cultural needs of the students in that setting.

Use of caring theory provides a foundation for how we practice as nurse educators even in the online environment. Specific theory concepts can provide the basis for our caring actions in the online educational setting. Furthermore, the online applications are teaching-learning examples founded on theory concepts that guide online caring actions. Table 6.1 presents online applications for the five Cs of caring, the theory of human caring (cybercaring), the nursing as caring model, and Leininger's theory of culture care diversity and universality, with associated select faculty caring actions.

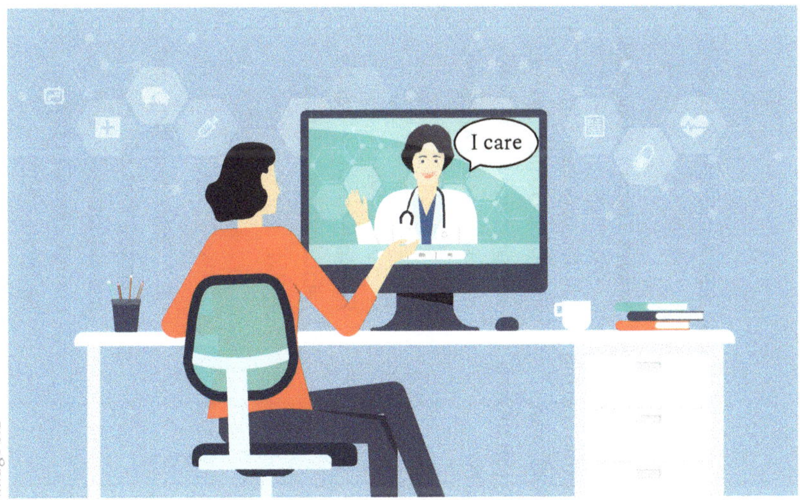

Image 6.1

TABLE 6.1 Caring Theories and Application to Online Teaching–Learning

Caring Theory	Select Theory Concepts	Online Teaching–Learning Application Examples	Select Online Faculty Caring Actions
Theory of human caring (Watson, 1985) and cybercaring (Sitzman & Watson, 2017)	Caritas process (CP) 1: Embrace altruistic values, and practice loving kindness with self and others (Watson, 1985)	CP 1: Digital Perspective: Kindness (Sitzman & Watson, 2017)	Social presence Friendliness and informal interaction in digital space (Sitzman & Watson, 2017)
	CP 4: Develop helping–trusting–caring relationships (Watson, 1985)	CP 4: Digital caring perspective: Developing helping–trusting–caring relationships in the digital world (Sitzman & Watson, 2017)	Design courses thoughtfully; provide quick, kind responses; allow for missteps in communication and practice forgiveness (Sitzman & Watson, 2017)
	CP 7: Share teaching and learning that address individual needs and comprehension styles (Watson, 1985)	CP 7: Digital caring perspective: Addressing individual needs for human connection (Sitzman & Watson, 2017)	One-on-one phone or video meetings; use voice recordings in place of text or emails; share new technology to meet individual student needs (Sitzman & Watson, 2017)

(Continued)

TABLE 6.1 (Continued)

Caring Theory	Select Theory Concepts	Online Teaching–Learning Application Examples	Select Online Faculty Caring Actions
Nursing as caring (Boykin & Schoenhofer, 2001)	Living and growing in caring; persons in academia support each other in caring; faculty support uniqueness of the individual and provide for an environment to grow and care; approach nursing situations with the patterns of knowing (Boykin & Schoenhofer, 2001)	Online course design	Navigation; use of accessibility and other LMS tools
		Online caring communication patterns; academic support	Netiquette; tone of text and audio; authentic online presence; caring communication; one-on-one Zoom meetings; use of course announcement feature; synchronous chat
		Learning nursing content online	Storytelling; threaded discussion boards; online collaborative assignments

(Continued)

TABLE 6.1 (Continued)

Caring Theory	Select Theory Concepts	Online Teaching–Learning Application Examples	Select Online Faculty Caring Actions
Human act of caring principles (Roach, 1992)	Nursing core is caring; humanism in education (Roach, 1992)	Online course design and implementation	Netiquette, navigation and alignment, use of accessibility and other LMS tools, use of current content in nursing
	Five Cs of caring: commitment, competence, conscience, compassion, confidence (Roach, 1992)	Faculty-to-student interactions	Course announcements; use of module 0; one-on-one interaction via phone and Zoom; use of synchronous chat rooms; timely, authentic feedback; responsiveness to communication
		Student-to-student interactions	Threaded discussion; collaboration, group work, teamwork, storytelling

(Continued)

TABLE 6.1 (Continued)

Caring Theory	Select Theory Concepts	Online Teaching–Learning Application Examples	Select Online Faculty Caring Actions
Leininger's theory of culture care diversity and universality (Leininger, 1991)	Theory supports care through three decision action modes: (1) preserve and maintain caring actions that work; (2) accommodate and negotiate on mutually agreed upon actions; (3) repattern and restructure caring actions based on mutual goals (Leininger, 1991; McFarland & Wehbe-Alamah, 2018)	Online caring communication patterns, academic support	Tone of text and audio, authentic online presence, netiquette
		Human interactions	Understand diverse needs of students
		Learning nursing content online	Incorporate content reflective of student diversity and healthcare population, storytelling, threaded discussion, use of diverse guest speakers

Caring in the Online Learning Environment: Essential Skills

Overview

The theories of caring guide nurse educators in caring actions in the online nursing education environment. Online nurse educator students learning the online faculty role must acquire the skills of caring, communication, and meaningful interaction from their place as online students in anticipation of "someday" teaching these virtual caring skills to *their* future students. One way that faculty can teach these essential online skills is to role model and provide examples of these attributes for online students in the virtual learning environment. A best practice for faculty is to use caring strategies in online courses and in everyday virtual interactions with students. Research about caring interactions and a discussion of how to operationalize caring actions follows.

Research and Online Caring Actions

Best practice in the online teaching environment starts with faculty awareness that online students perform better and have a greater chance of success when perceived as cared for by online faculty (Casey & Kroth, 2013; Cobb, 2009; Gazza & Hunker, 2014). Furthermore, online students desire faculty caring actions and social presence (Sitzman, 2010; Zajac & Lane, 2020). A scoping review of 38 articles in education literature about characteristics of high-quality online courses revealed several common areas related to faculty presence and support, such as response time; availability; well-defined directions; frequent posting; extending requests for student participation and engagement; and merging of faculty knowledge, online social presence, and teaching skills into the online learning environment (Wright et al., 2023).

Online faculty caring actions are exhibited through three major categories: (1) faculty social presence, (2) faculty immediacy, and (3) communication in the virtual learning environment. There is some overlap among the strategies discussed for each category of caring actions.

Faculty social presence is the process of exhibiting oneself as human in the online environment by expressing emotion and displaying social actions. Faculty presence is enhanced through the use of frequent and authentic communication. Showing emotion; addressing students by their preferred name; and using thoughtful, caring, positive, and authentic words are some examples of social presence (Wang, 2010; Zajac & Lang, 2020). Faculty social presence is regarded by online students as a form of caring (Zajac & Lane, 2020).

Faculty immediacy is similar to faculty presence and encompasses actions that represent verbal and nonverbal conduct, which may close the gap of perceived distance by the students. Examples of immediacy behaviors that personalize interactions in the learning environment are eye contact, vocal intonation and variation, facial expressions, relaxed body posture, and gestures. In the online environment, these examples are applied in faculty-created videos and audio presentations; course announcements; synchronous class video meetings, such as Zoom (http://zoom.com) and Skype (http://skype.com); and one-on-one video meetings and phone calls. Faculty immediacy is perceived as caring by online students (Huber et al., 2023) and can support healthy online interactions (Vlachopoulos, 2019).

Online *communication* is the construction of messages online that include a sender and a receiver and may include a feedback loop. Online caring communication involves the use of immediacy and social presence behaviors, such as addressing students by their preferred name and using thoughtful, caring, positive, and authentic words in audio, video, text announcements, email, and grading feedback. The three types of caring actions are associated with specific best practices to engage students, demonstrate caring, and foster online student success.

Caring Skills and Engagement

Students can engage in the learning environment in three ways: (1) faculty-to-student interaction, (2) student-to-student interaction, and (3) student-to-course interaction. The online teaching–learning setting offers opportunities for all three types of interaction; the use of caring skills enhances the experiences of the interactions. For example, with student-to-student interaction, students perceive better academic outcomes as online peer connections and interactions increase (Shatila, 2024). In addition, best caring practices have been adapted from face-to-face teaching methods to online education to enhance faculty-to-student and student-to-student interaction.

Faculty-to-Student and Student-to-Student Interactions

One example is the "seven best practices for teaching and learning" (Chickering & Gamson, 1987, p. 2), which are used extensively in higher education. The seven practices are:

1. Encourage contact between students and faculty.
2. Develop reciprocity and cooperation among students.
3. Use active learning techniques.
4. Give prompt feedback.
5. Emphasize time on task.
6. Communicate high expectations.
7. Respect diverse talents and ways of learning.

These seven practices have been further developed and adapted for online nursing education and provide direction for increasing faculty-to-student and student-to-student interactions (Koeckeritz et al., 2002). Of importance is that faculty-to-student interaction is perceived as caring by online students (Huber et al., 2023; Zajac & Lane, 2020). Table 6.2 presents examples of how to apply the seven best practices to online education, as adapted from Koeckeritz et al. (2002).

Student-to-Course Interactions

Online faculty enhance student-to-course interaction through academic support and investment in student success. Online caring actions to enhance course engagement include using a module 0 (see Chapter 4), providing a weekly overview via the LMS course announcement feature, offering to read sections of rough draft assignments and rewriting a few sentences as examples, including exemplar assignments, identifying students at risk and providing ongoing feedback, providing students with examples, providing detailed rubrics, keeping students on track by adding reminders for assignments and assessments, creating a tip sheet for success in the course, and including a weekly summary of the module/course topic. Several of these actions were discussed previously with ideas for course development and implementation in Chapters 2, 3, and 4. Online faculty develop these actions from a caring and empathetic perspective.

TABLE 6.2 Adapted Best Practices for Online Education

Chickering and Gamson's Original Seven Best Practices for Higher Education (1987)	Select Best Practice Actions for Online Teaching Learning
Encourage contact between students and faculty.	Email/course announcements Welcome students to class Practice netiquette Hold faculty virtual office hours Include synchronous chats or Zoom meetings Assign threaded discussions
Develop reciprocity and cooperation among students.	Establish discussion board groups and have students lead discussion Pair students for online activities and assignments
Use active learning techniques.	Use module 0 Set course expectations for participation Create interactive assignments Create online simulated experiences Assign student video presentations
Give prompt feedback.	Provide prompt, authentic feedback Adhere to grading deadlines
Emphasize time on task.	Publish due dates and timelines Provide announcement reminders Give prompts in module for upcoming assignments
Communicate high expectations.	Post academic integrity expectations Provide examples of expectations in online assignment feedback Provide detailed rubrics for online assignments
Respect diverse talents and ways of learning.	Identify learning styles Provide a variety of online teaching strategies Provide learner resources

Actions for online teaching adapted from: Koeckeritz, J., Malkiewicz, J., & Henderson, A. (2002). The seven principles of good practice: Application for online education in nursing. *Nurse Educator*, *27*(6), 283–287. https://doi.org/10.1097/00006223-200211000-00010

Communication: Strategies and Implementation

In the online setting, faculty should strive for interactive communication, which takes many forms, including writing/text, posts, announcements, email messages, and video and audio messages. The communication situations in the online teaching–learning environment may be faculty-to-student (and vice versa), student-to-student, and student-to-course. Faculty-to-student communication situations are discussed here. Faculty generate caring communication actions for a variety of reasons, such as standard practice, course communication, assignment feedback, or student triggers. Triggers are cues from online students that require a caring intervention by faculty; examples of triggers are lack of student participation in the discussion board or other course activity, decline in the quality of the student's work, submission of a late assignment, and/or student comments on Q&A discussion board or other course area that reveal confusion or frustration. A trigger prompts a caring communication response by faculty.

Principles of General Online Communication

Principles of caring communication include timeliness, quality, empathy, and authenticity. Faculty can demonstrate these attributes of caring communication and still maintain rigor in the online course. Key strategies for caring communication are to use the student's preferred name, identify triggers and respond, give individualized assignment feedback, post clarifying course announcements for difficult topics, be kind in communication responses and announcements, and respond to student emails within 24 hours (Zajac & Lane, 2020), or within the institution's established policy for email response. In addition, students should communicate using similar caring principles, such as kindness, clarity, timely response time, and use the faculty or other students' preferred names in the correspondence or post. The syllabus and module 0 are appropriate places to post the expectations for communication for both faculty and students.

Principles for Writing Email Responses and Assignment Feedback

Assignment feedback and email responses can convey caring and high expectations at the same time. For example, assignment feedback contains praise for good work as well as constructive suggestions. For an email response, the acronym GUARD reminds faculty of the components for writing a caring message that effectively communicates course standards and expectations; GUARD stands for Greeting, Understand, Answer, Reassure, and Dedication (Authement, 2019). Writing caring assignment feedback and composing GUARD emails takes time; however, the details in the communication demonstrate presence, exhibit caring without disregarding course policies, show investment in student success, and save time later.

In addition to written feedback, faculty can use video software located in the LMS and record comments to individual students about their discussion board posts and/or other assignments. One-on-one audio/video comments to students enhance faculty presence in the course; this feedback is in addition to completing the rubric associated with the assignment. Strategies specific to caring assignment feedback and email correspondence are provided in the *Teacher Tidbits*.

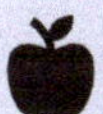

TEACHER TIDBITS FOR ASSIGNMENT FEEDBACK AND GRADING: USING CARING PRINCIPLES

- Grade assignments within one week of due date.
- Provide personalized and caring feedback.
- Address student by their preferred name.
- Use a positive opening sentence (e.g., "Good work on section 1 of the essay").
- Complement what resonates and then provide constructive feedback.
- If you are delayed in grading, communicate such to the students with a time frame.
- Late grading should be the exception, not the rule.

(Zajac & Lane, 2020)

Example for feedback for an online writing assignment:

Hi Kate,

Most of the required elements are present in the paper. Noted is the appropriate use of the literature to support your ideas. Good work! One suggestion that will strengthen the paper is to write in professional voice. For example, avoid the use of slang terms. The online writing center at (*give the link*) provides assistance through virtual appointments with students. I am also available to read paragraph drafts of assignments. Please refer to the rubric for specific grade details and reach out if you have questions.

—Dr. Faculty

TEACHER TIDBITS FOR CARING EMAIL PRINCIPLES: USE THE ACRONYM GUARD

- Greeting: Address the student personally.
- Understand: Acknowledge the concern or issue.
- Answer: Provide information and resources.
- Reassure: Provide encouragement.
- Dedication: be available

(Authement, 2019; Authement & Dormire, 2020)

Email from student:
I just reviewed my grade and your comments for my presentation. I think my grade is too low. I worked very hard on this assignment. I find it difficult to work, attend school online, and then have a presentation due the same week along with the discussion board posts. It is too much for one class. I think my grades should be higher in this course.

—Jim

Faculty response using GUARD:

Hi Jim,

Thank you for your email and for sharing your concerns. The combination of work and school when enrolled in an online program can be challenging from a time management perspective. In the syllabus, you will find a table with a suggested number of hours to spend on each assignment every week. I posted the date for the presentation assignment at the beginning of the term in the LMS course and in the syllabus on page 6. One suggestion is to work a little each week on large course assignments. In the future, the online tutors may be helpful to you; they can be reached at (*provide link*). Please review the comments and feedback that I provided in the gradebook and on the rubric—click on the feedback link within the grade book. I am willing to review a draft of assignments prior to submission. My goal is to see you succeed. Email me if you have questions.

Sincerely, Dr. Faculty

SHOW WHAT YOU KNOW ASSIGNMENT

Create a sample email using GUARD in response to the following online student email:

Hi Dr. Faculty,

I looked at my grade that you gave me on the short paper leadership assignment and I would like the opportunity to resubmit the assignment. I see where I missed the parts of the rubric. In my other class, we are allowed to revise and resubmit assignments. I hope that is the same rule in your course. Please let me know. I am finding that the expectations for this course are somewhat high. From, Your Student.

Faculty response (assume that faculty do not permit resubmissions of assignments):

____

____

Faculty Social Presence and Immediacy: Strategies and Implementation

Social Presence

Many strategies are available to demonstrate presence and humanness, some of which overlap with strategies previously discussed for caring communication. Caring actions for faculty social presence include sharing some personal information in the faculty bio for the course, such as hobbies, career experience, and capability with the course content (see Chapter 4). In addition, other online social presence ideas are to provide a welcome letter for the course; identify ways to reach the professor; participate in the discussion board; and, if possible, respond to all students' first posts. Other ideas are to offer course guidance; regular announcements that contain reminders and updates; callouts to specific students for course participation; general course check-ins via announcements or short videos; and chapter highlights, wrap-ups, and summaries. One time-saving feature is to have a file of prewritten generic course highlights, summaries, wrap-ups, and announcements, and then adding a few lines to make it specific to the present group of students.

Faculty Immediacy

Faculty immediacy closes the perceived distance between students and faculty in the online environment. The immediacy strategies, some of which overlap with faculty presence ideas, include use of video meetings, video and audio course content material, phone calls, video announcements, emails, and presenting as authentic self. For example, be authentic and humble when you correspond or post, admit when you (the faculty) have made a mistake, and state how you will correct the mistake. It is important to be flexible in online courses and respond to students when triggers are apparent. Use of phrases such as "Just checking in…" or "I noticed that…" may assist with email conversations when students' issues are noted. Students ranked the top three characteristics for online faculty who display immediacy as (1) providing timely communication, (2) offering academic support, and (3) presenting an empathetic presence (Huber et al., 2023). The use of video cannot be understated. A faculty-produced video lets students know that you are present in the course.

Novice nurse educators can learn about caring actions, social presence, and immediacy behaviors from experienced nurse educators as well. Read the *Experiences from the Virtual World* (Box 6.1) for an interview between an online nurse educator, Dr. Lauren Theuerling, DNP, APRN, and the book author about caring for students and exhibiting social presence and immediacy. The interview responses reinforce findings from the literature and best practices from online and nursing education experts.

BOX 6.1 Experiences from the Virtual World

Question: How do you incorporate caring and presence into the online teaching/learning environment?

Dr. Theuerling: There are many opportunities: I make sure that I provide a welcome email; I use professional but friendly terms in my emails to students. I let them know that I am always available for questions. It is important to be open for being contacted by students. In addition, I send [email] course updates for the week which include helpful hints and resources, and I offer examples. When students reach out to me, I offer reassurance and support them. Other ways that I show caring are to use voiceover PowerPoint presentations. I also tap into [specific] learning styles with different teaching strategies. To keep current, I use up-to-date content and resources and use guest speakers to make the online course "more real" [applicable].

Question: What are your perceptions of the benefits of caring actions in the online environment?

Dr. Theuerling: Students have busy schedules and their lives include graduate school, multiple roles, and responsibilities. They get their online coursework done when time is available and they like online courses for the flexibility. They can easily access online school, however, asynchronous [modes of delivery] can be tricky for them. Students need to be self-motivated and use their own time when available so sometimes attending school can be under the radar. This is why faculty caring and communication with students are vital.

Question: What are some challenges or barriers to online teaching?

Dr. Theuerling: Communication can be a challenge due to lack of face-to-face interaction. For course development one must maintain professional standards even in the online environment. Another challenge is the faculty learning curve for understanding the LMS platform and upgrades as well as learning the apps for online teaching/learning.

Another factor is appreciating that there are different ways that students learn so I consider different ways of presenting course material; faculty can use different types of creative strategies. Groupwork may be challenging for some students due to living in different time zones, which must be considered. For some faculty and students, technical glitches can be a barrier.

Question: How do you convey caring in a virtual educational setting?

Dr. Theuerling: I suggest adding a faculty bio that contains something personal. I also send an email if student work is subpar. In the email I offer assistance and state, "I would like you to be successful." Faculty can be caring and have boundaries but be flexible, for example, the consideration of assignment extensions.

Additional Application of Online Caring Actions

Use of the Course Map

For novice online faculty, noting specific caring actions on the course map during the planning and design phase of the course may be helpful. For examples of caring actions appropriate for week 1 of an online course, refer to the Caring Actions section in the course map below. Recall that the course map was created in Chapter 2 and then updated in Chapters 3, 4, and 5 (Box 6.2).

BOX 6.2 Course Map Week 1 with Caring Actions Added

Name of course: Translation and Utilization of Evidence for Nursing Practice		
Units	**Unit 1**	**Unit 2**
Unit title/topic	Review and appraisal of the literature	
End-of-program outcome(s) (EPO)	EPO 3: Utilize systematic processes to appraise evidence for application to nursing practice.	
Course objective(s) (CO)	CO 1: Critically appraise nursing and healthcare literature and clinical guidelines.	
Unit objective(s) (UO)	By the end of this unit, the student will: UO 1: Differentiate between the types of literature. UO 2: List the levels of literature evidence. UO 3: Identify the strength and quality of a variety of healthcare literature. UO 4: Appraise a variety of literature, including quantitative, qualitative, gray literature.	
Assignment/ activity (List one or more activities for each week or unit, as appropriate. Label the unit objective that aligns with the assignment/ activity.)	• Review a short video presentation about literature appraisal. (UO 3, UO 4) • Read Chapters 1 through 4 in the textbook. (UO 1–4) • Review articles X, Y, Z as examples of different types of literature/ evidence. (UO 2) • Appraise one research journal article and summarize. (UO 2–4) • Post responses to the following question in the discussion board. (OU 1–4)	

Units	Unit 1	Unit 2
Assessment/ evaluation (List one or more assessments for each week or unit, as appropriate. Label with the unit objective that aligns with the assessment activity.)	Graded discussion board (OU 1–4) (See discussion board rubric.) Appraisal assessment: Appraisal and summary of research journal article (see rubric). (UO 2–4)	
High-impact practice	Add the research article appraisal and summary assessment to the ePortfolio. (UO 1–4)	
Principles of universal design	Add items related to accessibility here: • Run accessibility checker for documents, presentations, web pages; provide alt text and descriptions as needed. • Audio and video include caption and text capture.	
	• Provide table headings. • Use links to click and connect. • Avoid the use of bold and color to enhance meaning. • Layout is simple and easy to navigate.	
Inclusive design	• Check for inclusive language. • Check tone and rhetoric of course. • Adopt an inclusive syllabus (check policies, descriptions, and course requirements).	
Tools and apps for online teach-ing and learning	• Add tools/apps used in Unit 1.	

Units	Unit 1	Unit 2
Caring actions (examples for Week 1)	• Provide welcome letter/course announcement. • Acknowledge students in the introduction DB posts; create a first post interaction. • Use faculty-created videos for welcome, content, or content clarification. • Provide chapter highlights, wrap-ups, or summaries, either by course announcement or short video. • Post grade turnaround times and response times. • Grade the first week DB and journal appraisal assignment using authentic, timely feedback.	

SHOW WHAT YOU KNOW ASSIGNMENT

Directions: Add additional examples of caring actions in the green space for Unit 1/Module 1 that represent authentic communication, faculty online social presence, and immediacy. Share ideas with your peers.

Name of course: Translation and Utilization of Evidence for Nursing Practice

Unit	Unit 1	Unit 2
Unit title/topic		
End-of-program outcome(s) (EPO)		
Course objective(s) (CO)		

Unit	Unit 1	Unit 2
Unit objective(s) (UO)		
Assignment/activity (List one or more activities for each week or unit, as appropriate. Label the unit objective that aligns with the assignment/activity.)		
Assessment/evaluation (List one or more assessments for each week or unit, as appropriate. Label with the unit objective that aligns with the assessment activity.)		
High-impact practice		
Principles of universal design		
Inclusive design		
Online tools/apps		
Caring actions (examples for course week 1)	Add examples of caring actions that represent authentic communication, faculty online social presence, and immediacy.	

Troubleshooting

Best practices for appropriate online caring communication depend on adequate technology, faculty knowledge, and good course design. While faculty have good intentions to employ caring communicative actions, glitches can and will occur. Broad recommendations to overcome barriers that interfere with caring communication are to troubleshoot the issue early and identify solutions to rectify the glitch. See "Glitches and Ditches" for a list of suggestions for troubleshooting specific online communication glitches.

GLITCHES AND DITCHES: TROUBLESHOOTING

Glitches and Ditches	Troubleshooting Suggestions
The intent of the communication may be lost in email or text messages.	Use positive words, be enthusiastic, and always be professional. Consider the use of emojis, when appropriate.
There are fewer opportunities for faculty-to-student and student-to-student interaction in the online environment if faculty are not intentional.	Plan opportunities for online caring interactions ahead of course implementation. Use a course map and add caring actions. Write down ideas for interaction when you think of them. Use resources (see Chapter Resources).
Technology may interfere with video or audio transmission in a course.	Have a "plan B" for synchronous sessions. When tech glitches occur, either on the student or faculty side, be flexible with timelines and deadlines.

Glitches and Ditches	Troubleshooting Suggestions
Phone calls inhibit the ability to see facial expressions.	Use a positive tone. Speak clearly. Discuss student accomplishments. Provide constructive feedback. Offer to help when appropriate.
Students may want to hide or be invisible in the online teaching–learning setting.	Provide opportunities for teamwork and/or group work. Include graded interactive assignments such as discussion boards, peer reviews, and debates.
Online communication mistakes happen.	Take ownership. Promptly correct mistakes. Be forgiving and/or apologize depending on the situation.

Conclusion

Caring theories for nursing drive the educational practice of caring and are also well suited for the online teaching–learning environment. Educational research supports caring practices in the online environment as important for student success and satisfaction. Faculty demonstrate caring actions through appropriate online communication, faculty social presence, and immediacy. Caring actions are vital to student-to-student interactions, student-to-faculty interactions, and student-to-course interactions. Online faculty can use a course map to plan intentional caring actions. In addition, faculty are prepared to troubleshoot communication and technology issues when they occur. Caring is fundamental to the practice of the art of nursing and therefore a necessary component of online nursing education.

TAKE 5

List five take-away points from Chapter 6.

What did you learn?

1.
2.
3.
4.
5.

What additional information do you need to understand the concepts? See the Chapter Resources for additional material.

CHAPTER ACTIVITIES

1. Complete the two "Show What You Know Assignments:
    - Compose the GUARD email.
    - Add caring actions to the course map.
    - Both activities will benefit the course design.
2. Self-care check-in. What is your progress with the self-care activity? Do you have time to engage in the two self-care activities on a regular basis? If not, consider committing to just one activity. Is your accountability person still the same? Are you checking in with them regularly? What barriers, if any, prevent you from engaging in self-care? Keep journaling your activities, note your feelings, identify barriers to engaging in self-care, and add solutions for overcoming the barriers. Keep up the good work! Remember that a little self-care is better than none at all.

JOURNAL EXAMPLE

Self-Care Activity 1:									
Date									
Feelings									
Barriers									
Other Notes									
Self-Care Activity 2:									
Date									
Feelings									
Barriers									
Other Notes									

CHAPTER RESOURCES

1. *Faculty Focus* is a website dedicated to faculty. *Faculty Focus* publishes three articles each week written by instructors, teachers, instructional designers, and others from around the world.

   https://www.facultyfocus.com

2. International Association for Human Caring (IAHA; https://www.humancaring.org) is an organization that welcomes people from "all cultures and backgrounds and professional disciplines to explore, discover, share knowledge and experiences related to Caring. The mission of IAHA is to create positive Caring in healthcare and beyond" (para. 1).

   https://www.humancaring.org/page-18114

REFERENCES

Authement, R. (2019, July 8-12). *GUARD for email roadmap to online teaching success.* 29th Annual Nurse Educator Conference in the Rockies, Vail, Colorado.

Authement, R. S., & Dormire, S. L. (2020). Introduction to the online nursing education best practices guide. *SAGE Open Nursing, 6*, 2377960820937290. https://doi.org/10.1177/2377960820937290

Boykin, A., & Schoenhofer, S. (2001). *Nursing as caring: A model of transforming practice.* NLN Press.

Casey, R., & Kroth, M. (2013). Learning to develop presence online: Experienced faculty perspectives. *Journal of Adult Education, 24*(2), 104–223.

Chickering, A., & Gamson, Z. (1987). Seven principles for good practice in undergraduate education. *AAHE Bulletin,* 3–7. Retrieved from https://files.eric.ed.gov/fulltext/ED282491.pdf

Cobb, S. C. (2009). Social presence and online learning: A current view from a research perspective. *Journal of Interactive Online Learning, 8*(3), 241–254.

Gazza, E., & Hunker, D. (2014). Facilitating student retention in online graduate nursing education programs: A review of the literature. *Nurse Education Today, 43*, 1125–1129. doi:10.1016/j.nedt.2014.01.010

Hayne, A. N., Schlosser, S. P., & McDaniel, G. S. (2020). A caring model for nursing education. *International Journal of Nursing Education Scholarship, 17*(1), 1–14. https://doi-org/10.1515/ijnes-2019-0072

Huber, T., Zajac, L., O'Connell, K., Robinson, D., & Lane, A. (2023). Student perceptions of nursing faculty immediacy: Caring actions for accelerated online courses. *Journal of Educators Online*, 20(3), 1–13. https://doi.org/10.9743/jeo.2023.20.3.1

Koeckeritz, J., Malkiewicz, J., & Henderson, A. (2002). The seven principles of good practice: Application for online education in nursing. *Nurse Educator, 27*(6), 283–287. https://doi.org/10.1097/00006223-200211000-00010

Leininger, M. M. (1991). *Culture care diversity & universality: A theory of nursing.* National League for Nursing.

Leininger, M. M., & McFarland, M. R. (2005). *Culture care diversity & universality: A worldwide nursing theory.* Jones & Bartlett.

Merriam-Webster. (2024). Definition of caring. https://www.merriam-webster.com/dictionary/caring

McFarland, M. R., & Wehbe-Alamah, H. B. (2018). *Leininger's transcultural nursing: Concepts, theories, research & practice.* (4th ed.). McGraw Hill Education.

Roach, S. (1992). *The human act of caring: A blueprint for the health professions.* (Revised ed.). Canadian Hospital Association Press.

Shatila, S. (2024). Not alone when I'm feeling stressed: Online adult learner connection and retention. *Adult Education Quarterly, 74*(1) 43–61. https://doi.org/10.1177/07417136231184570

Sitzman, K. (2010). Student-preferred caring behaviors for online nursing education. *Nursing Education Perspectives, 31*(3), 172–178.

Sitzman, K., & Watson, J. (2017). *Watson's caring in the digital world.* Springer.

Skype. (2024). *Meeting software.* Microsoft Corporation. https://www.skype.com/en/free-conference-call/

Vlachopoulos, D., & Makri, A. (2019). Online communication and interaction in distance higher education: A framework study of good practice. *International Review of Education, 65*, 605–632. https://doi.org/10.1007/s11159-019-09792-3

Wang, H. (2010, February, 18). Eight ways to increase social presence in your online classes. *Faculty Focus.* https://www.facultyfocus.com/articles/online-education/online-course-delivery-and-instruction/eight-ways-to-increase-social-presence-in-your-online-classes/

Watson, J. (1985). *Nursing: Human science and human care.* National League for Nursing.

Watson, J. (1997). The theory of human caring: Retrospective and prospective. *Nursing Science Quarterly, 10*(1), 49–52. https://doi.org/10.1177/089431849701000114

Wright, A., Carley, C. Alarakyia-Jivani, R., & Nizamuddin, S. (2023). Features of high-quality online courses in higher education: A scoping review. *Online Learning Journal, 27*(1), 46–70. https://doi.org/10.24059/olj.v27i1.3411

Zajac, L., & Lane, A. (2020). Student perceptions of faculty presence and caring in accelerated online courses. *Quarterly Review of Distance Education, 21*(2), 67–88.

Zoom. (2024). *Zoom products: Meetings[software].* Zoom Video Communications. https://www.zoom.com/en/products/virtual-meetings/?_ga=2.3899314.369901025.1709005968- 1621043773.1698414870/

Credits

CHAPTER 7

The Essentials of Diversity, Equity, and Inclusion in the Online Classroom

"Diversity is the mix. Inclusion is making the mix work."

—ANDRES TAPIA
(GLOBAL DIVERSITY AND INCLUSION STRATEGIST/LEADER)

TERMS TO KNOW

bias in education: Unfair or different treatment of students or other persons due to a diversity characteristic or other characteristics (see examples under *diversity in education*).

diversity in education: The variety of individual and group characteristics presented in people. Examples in education could be personality, life experiences, and learning styles. Group and/or social characteristics include race/ethnicity, age, class, gender, sexual orientation, country of origin, physical or cognitive abilities, as well as cultural, political, religious, or other affiliations that students and faculty present with to the teaching–learning environment.

equality in education: That all students get the same educational resources and support despite their individual needs.

equity education: Providing the necessary resources and opportunities with consideration for each student's circumstances so they can reach their highest academic and social capability.

explicit bias: A conscious preference or aversion toward a person or group of people that results from deliberate thoughts that we can identify and communicate with others.

inclusion in education: Comprises the individual's and academic institution's actions that foster acceptance, respect, and value for every person. Inclusion ensures that all members are provided the benefits and opportunities they are entitled to. Inclusion supports a sense of belonging.

microaggression: Can be conscious or unconscious subtle acts of discrimination against members of a marginalized group. In education, it could be exclusion from a group or derogatory comments about one's diversity characteristic.

sense of belonging in education: The outcome of inclusion; is tied to student learning and success.

unconscious or implicit bias in education: Unfair treatment and/or thoughts or feelings about students or other persons that occur outside of conscious awareness.

Chapter Overview and Objectives

This chapter presents issues related to diversity, equity, and inclusion (DEI) in nursing and healthcare education in the online teaching-learning environment. Current research and nursing profession standards that support DEI initiatives in nursing education are presented. Learners identify acts of bias and microaggressions in the online educational setting. Nurse educator strategies for creating an inclusive and safe virtual learning environment are reviewed for application to online course design.

In this chapter, the learner will:

1. Differentiate terminology associated with diversity, equity, and inclusion efforts in higher education.
2. Identify equity, diversity, inclusion, and social justice issues that create barriers to online education.
3. Recognize acts of microaggression in the online learning environment.
4. Assess one's own bias and actions that may deter effective teaching/learning.
5. Create strategies to promote safe, equitable, and just online learning environments.

Introduction to Diversity, Equity, and Inclusion (DEI) in Higher Education

As online programs in higher education grow, so does the population of diverse students (National Center for Education Statistics [NCES], 2021). Generally, students associate nursing and nursing school with high stress (Fruh et al., 2021; He et al., 2018; Zhuang-Shuang & Hasson, 2020); this stress in nursing education also applies to the online educational environment (He et al., 2018). Additionally, students who are ethnically and racially diverse face unique stressors and challenges to learning within a dominant culture of higher education. Ethnically and racially diverse students face acts of bias, microaggression, racism, inequity, and incivility in everyday spaces within institutions of learning (Lee & Hopson, 2019; Miles et al., 2021; Pusey-Reid et al., 2022), including the face-to-face nursing education environment (Iheduru-Anderson & Wahi, 2021; Jennings et al., 2024; Zajac, 2015; Zajac & Benton-Lee, 2023). Diverse students who learn online are faced with situations that may induce faculty biases, for example, the use of a student profile picture, connection to an ethnic name, and the understanding or lack of understanding of the academic environment (Benander & Rankey, 2021) and acts of microaggression (Zajac & Benton-Lee, 2023). In addition, diverse students may have a diminished sense of belonging to the online academic setting (Taylor et al., 2023).

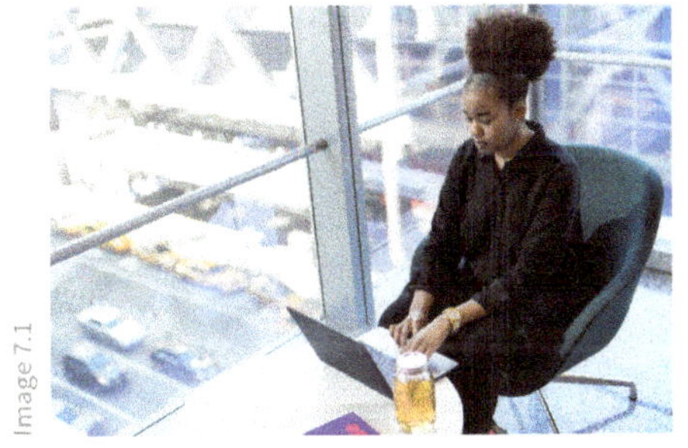
Image 7.1

In 2004, the report *Missing Persons: Minorities in the Health Professions* called for measures to decrease educational barriers for diverse healthcare students with the goal of expanding the number of diverse healthcare providers to match the diversity of the population (Sullivan, 2004). The imbalance in the number of diverse healthcare providers compared to the population still exists today. Nurse leaders appeal for initiatives to increase and retain diverse nurses in *The Future of Nursing 2020–2030: Charting a Path to Achieve Health Equity Report;* the report directs nurse educators to promote inclusivity and remove barriers, provide holistic support to students, and address institutional inequities (National Academies of Sciences, Engineering, & Medicine [NASEM], 2021). All nurse faculty, including those who teach online, are compelled to create a safe and inclusive classroom that is free of bias and other negative behaviors, including racism, microaggressions, and discrimination.

Actions That Disrupt Safe Educational Spaces

Bias and Discrimination in Online Education

Acts of bias, discrimination, and microaggressions create barriers to equity in online education and disrupt learning spaces. Bias in online education takes several forms; it can be implicit (hidden) or explicit (obvious) and impact education equity. For example, diverse online students may perceive that their life experiences or input are unseen or not valued (Crutchfied et al., 2022). In addition, diverse students may experience overt exclusion from White student groups (Miles et al., 2020). Other examples of bias and discrimination include a lack of racial and ethnic diversity in teaching materials, such as images in slide or video presentations, and the absence of diversity in course content, textbooks, and authors (Benander & Rankey, 2021; Brooks & Grady, 2022). A gender and ethnicity bias study in the online learning environment found that White male students were more likely to receive responses from course faculty than White female students and Asian males; in the same study, White female students were more likely to receive responses from their peers than White male students (Baker et al., 2022). These experiences of bias and discrimination can interfere with a student's sense of belonging in the academic environment (Taylor et al., 2023).

Racial Microaggressions

One form of discrimination is microaggressions, defined as offensive and/or threatening verbal or nonverbal behaviors toward diverse and or marginalized groups; the offending person may be unconscious of the microaggressive actions (Sue, 2010; Sue & Spanierman, 2020).

Racial microaggressions are the "communication of hostile, derogatory, or negative racial slights and insults to people of color" (Sue, 2010, p. 29). Sue and others classify microaggressions as microinsults, microassaults, or microinvalidations (Sue et al., 2007; Sue et al., 2008). The microaggression categories represented by race are (1) racial microinsults, which are comments or actions directed at someone's racial, ethnic, or cultural identity, often committed unconsciously; (2) racial microassaults, which are hurtful, harassing actions that range from name-calling to avoidance due to race, which may be subtle or overt; and (3) racial microinvalidations, which are actions that invalidate a diverse person's lived experience or truth (Sue, 2010). Racial microaggressions happen in institutions of higher learning and are associated with health consequences and other untoward effects for diverse students (Ackerman-Barger et al., 2020; Lee & Hopson, 2019; Melendez & Thompson, 2020) and can disrupt the sense of belonging in the academic setting (Taylor et al., 2023).

Racial Microaggressions in the Online Environment

Examples of racial microaggressions in the online environment include derogatory comments in the discussion board, lack of diverse teaching materials and strategies, disregard for student posts, and general invalidation actions (Zajac & Benton-Lee 2023). In addition, diverse students may carry over past traumatic educational experiences of previous microaggressions from either traditional or online settings to the present learning environment. Another example of microaggression could be the use of a profile picture in the online course; faculty ask or require students to introduce themselves, which at the very least could include name, location, and a profile picture. Online faculty should weigh the pros and cons of requiring a student to post a profile picture that could make a student vulnerable to acts of microaggression; students should have a choice when asked to post a profile picture in a course (Zajac & Benton-Lee, 2023). See Box 7.1 for comments and stories from a descriptive qualitative study about the student experience of microaggressions in the online environment.

BOX 7.1 Microaggression Experiences: Comments from Diverse Online Nursing Students

- **Carryover from past traumatic educational experience:**

"I think sometimes I feel like I have to say more to make it look like I'm more educated, and that could just be something I feel… I haven't had anyone say anything to me, but I just feel like I have to put more into my discussion posts [and] on my papers because I feel like there is always a stigma."

- **Use of photo or profile picture in an online course:**

"I feel like, sometimes, when it comes to African Americans, our names can be associated with preconceived perceptions because they aren't traditional names. I feel like without seeing a profile picture you won't [assume student XX is a] ghetto-type person or aggressive type. [Without the profile picture], you get a different association of me."

- **Online course microinvalidation:**

"Each time that I've posted an introduction, they [faculty] want us to… comment or message on two other people. I don't think anyone's ever messaged on mine, and I actually have a really close friend who lives in my neighborhood… in the same program, and she's White and has several messages on hers like 'It's nice to meet you,' you know. No one has honed in on mine."

- **Microinsult during an online course group project:**

"… not sure if it had to do with anything about me being Hispanic/Latina, but, um, that's, the only thing I can say it was a little micro-aggressive where nobody else was focused on the other students [in my group], but the students were focusing on me getting my job done which I had not shown any signs that it was not going to get achieved."

Adapted from: Zajac, L. & Benton-Lee. J. (2023). Microaggressions: Experiences of diverse graduate nursing students in online education. *Journal of Transcultural Nursing, 34*(4), 301–309. https://doi.org/10.1177/10436596231166043

Online Faculty Assessment of Bias and Actions for Change

Caring presence was discussed in detail in Chapter 6 as being associated with student success. In fact, a study about online faculty presence revealed that 91 percent of online students believe the presence or absence of caring on the part of the online instructor influenced success in the course (Zajac & Lane, 2020). Caring and presence in the online environment extends to the responsibility for attending to bias and discriminatory behaviors that may interfere with inclusive or equitable learning environments and a sense of belonging for diverse students. Little has been published about how to operationalize strategies to support students from a DEI perspective in the online environment, which supports the need for more faculty to learn how to integrate inclusive approaches in the virtual classroom. In reality, online faculty may struggle with inclusion, diversity, equity, and inclusion issues in online education. A study by Miller et al. (2023) found that faculty report more comfort with inclusion and educational access and are less comfortable about diversity and equity in the online classroom. Although more education research is needed in these areas, actions begin with fostering faculty–student interactions and caring about the students.

Self-Reflection

Faculty can take action to foster a safe, inclusive, equitable online learning environment through self-reflection on bias and intentional actions to increase understanding of diverse students' experiences. The American Association of Colleges of Nursing (AACN) urges nurse educators to self-reflect on bias behaviors that could interfere with an inclusive, equitable learning environment for diverse students (AACN, 2017). Crutchfield and others (2022) recommend self-reflection by asking the following questions about bias using a self-reflective manner:

> What biases do I hold about race? Am I biased against virtual education? How might these biases impact my course development and delivery? Do I understand and acknowledge the ways in which my own racial and ethnic identity impacts how I see the world? (p. 748).

The National Education Association (NEA) offers suggestions to address personal implicit bias (https://www.nea.org/recognizing-your-biases). Implicit bias is when one is not consciously aware of the bias behavior or actions. The suggestions from the NEA (2024) start with the self-awareness of thoughts and feelings about biases and taking the time to view each person as an individual rather than from a particular group. After increasing awareness, additional suggestions include:

1. Be conscious of and question your decisions [and actions]. Be kind to students and be an example for understanding.
2. Educate yourself; use available resources and bias assessment tools such as the free one found at Project Implicit. https://implicit.harvard.edu/implicit/. Take the Implicit Bias assessment and reflect on your findings. Use the results of the assessment to bring awareness to the biases in one's behavior.
3. Work with systems and organizations to reduce bias while you work on the implicit bias within yourself. Be honest that there is implicit bias in everyone.
4. Increase exposure to people who are different than you; step out of your comfort zone to increase interactions with others to decrease any stereotypes. Be intentional about inclusiveness. (NEA, 2024)

For more information about bias and bias assessment tools, see the Chapter 7 Resources.

Implementing Strategies for Equitable and Inclusive Online Learning Spaces

Chapter 3 discussed strategies for designing courses with inclusivity in mind and offered the following strategies: ensure student access to technology, commit to diversity and inclusion, include images and content that reflect diversity to course content, foster faculty-to-student and student-to-student interaction, recognize bias in self and others, create inclusive syllabi, and connect students to support services (Benander & Rankey, 2021; Brooks & Grady, 2022; Zajac & Benton-Lee, 2023). This chapter presents ways to implement several of these strategies to ensure an inclusive, safe online learning environment.

Assess for and Remove Bias in Course Content

Jennings et al. (2024) suggest the use of a bias checklist to evaluate nursing coursework for identity and content bias across the 14 bias domains of gender, image, sexual orientation, mental illness, racial, age, interprofessional, poverty, disability, weight, prisoner, clinical vignettes, religious, and immigrant. Course documents, images, text (articles, book chapters), videos, and podcasts are all forms of course materials that can be evaluated quickly using the Upstate Bias Checklist (UBCL). The original checklist was developed by Caruso Brown et al. (2019) and is available in the public domain. See the appendix at the end of the chapter for more information about how to access the checklist.

Additional strategies assist faculty to engage more equitably and to decrease bias in an online course. One recommendation is to remove student pictures and names for anonymous grading from the course to create an equitable online classroom (Baker et al., 2022; Lin & Kennette, 2021). Another strategy is to create a welcoming online course inclusive of all students so that the space feels safe and allows for a multitude of voices, opinions, and student identities (Crutchfield et al., 2022). Faculty establish the virtual safe space through open online dialogue, discussion about acceptable behavior, and providing students the freedom to express ideas. Additional recommendations are to include course materials, images, presentations, and content experts/authors and guest speakers that represent the diversity of the population. Faculty can learn from minority students and take time to listen to their stories, be an empathetic presence, provide opportunities to increase online engagement between faculty and students, operationalize the components of an inclusive syllabus (see Chapter 6), and teach nursing content inclusive of the various healthcare needs of diverse populations.

Address Microaggression in the Online Environment

Faculty can add additional online classroom norms that address DEI to the list of course rules and netiquette located in the course

"Start Here" module. Faculty must adopt a zero-tolerance policy for microaggressive actions. Violation of classroom norms and/or the occurrence of microaggression should be dealt with promptly. Review the example of a faculty intervention for a microaggression situation in the *Teacher Tidbits*. An engaged online faculty should be attentive to inappropriate online behavior. Another recommendation is to take time in the course when appropriate to teach and provide information about what actions constitute microaggression, especially in the online environment.

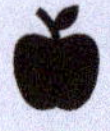

TEACHER TIDBITS: ADDRESSING MICROAGGRESSIONS IN THE ONLINE CLASSROOM

- **Example microaggression**: A student's current job involves delivering medical equipment to various clinics around the city. In a discussion board post visible to everyone in the course, the student posted a statement about being at a clinic in a rough neighborhood in the inner city. (This is an example of a microinsult.)
- **Faculty response:** The faculty responds in a one-on-one virtual setting with the student. The response can be written or verbal: "I have a concern with your post in which you referred to a rough neighborhood in the inner city. As per our class norms, students are to avoid using terms that can be interpreted as demeaning. A description of a rough neighborhood is an individual perception from one's lived experience, and it may be different from another's lived experience of work and home. Terms such as 'rough neighborhood' or 'inner city' could be perceived negatively. Course norms in this class require us to be sensitive to how we use terms. A microaggression can be in the form of a comment, which, although may be unintentional, may have negative connotations and be hurtful to a person or specific group. Please reach out to me if you have questions or concerns."

Ongoing Faculty Work

Research demonstrates that microaggressions are experienced by diverse students. The continuing needs of diverse students warrant faculty attention and efforts to create an environment free from microaggressions. Faculty can mitigate microaggressions in areas such as emails, student presentations, and discussion boards by adhering to the no-tolerance policy and taking action when microaggressions occur. Other efforts include the development of additional strategies, further research, and actions to diminish microaggression and foster learning in the virtual setting. And finally, inviting a peer faculty who is skilled in online DEI strategies for appraisal of your online course may yield additional ways to create an inclusive milieu.

SHOW WHAT YOU KNOW ASSIGNMENT

1. What strategies can you use to include student voices in discussion and presenting material? How can you encourage students to use all of their language skills in assignments, whether multilingual research or visual or spoken presentations?
2. How can course materials such as presentations, textbooks, and activities reflect the diversity of the students and/or the population that the students care for?
3. How could you apply your values about diversity when creating your course assessments?

Adapted from: Kumar, R., & Refaei, B. (2021). *Equity and inclusion in higher education: Strategies for teaching*. University of Cincinnati Press.

Conclusion

In education, faculty have an obligation to provide all students with the tools and the safe learning space to support success. The same actions are expected of online faculty. Diverse students face unique challenges in higher education that require attention. The first step is for faculty to reflect on their own biases, and then implement best practice strategies to ensure equity and safety in the online learning environment. DEI goes beyond the online classroom. Faculty advocacy extends to all virtual places in higher education institutions, including the library, student services, writing centers, inclusive instructional technologies, and instructional design departments (Miller et al., 2023). Faculty can request professional development about DEI for themselves, instructional designers, and other university employees. Together, we all can advocate for an optimal educational experience for diverse online students.

TAKE 5

List five take-away points from Chapter 7.

What did you learn?

1.
2.
3.
4.
5.

What additional information do you need to understand the concepts? See the Chapter Resources for additional material.

CHAPTER ACTIVITIES

1. Complete the Implicit Bias activity found at https://implicit.harvard.edu/implicit/takeatest.html. Write down any thoughts or feelings that you have about the exercise.
2. **Sharing on Caring:** Keep journaling your self-care activities. Note your feelings, identify barriers to engaging in self-care, and add solutions for overcoming the barriers. Keep up the good work! Remember that a little self-care is better than none at all.
3. Consider a course you are enrolled in or teaching. Use the Update Bias Checklist (see link under the Chapter Resources) to assess for bias in course documents, for example,

presentations, reading assignments, case studies, videos, and images.

4. Complete the "Show What You Know Assignment."

CHAPTER RESOURCES

1. Upstate Bias Checklist and Manual: https://u.osu.edu/ocscom/curriculum/instructional-design/upstate-bias-checklist/
2. Find bias testing and free versions of the tests are available at the Project Implicit website: https://implicit.harvard.edu/implicit/
3. NEA Toolkit: Implicit Bias, Microaggressions, and Stereotypes Resources: https://www.nea.org/resource-library/implicit-bias-microaggressions-and-stereotypes-resources
4. American Bar Association People with Disabilities and Implicit Bias: https://www.americanbar.org/groups/diversity/disabilityrights/resources/implicit_bias/
5. Project Implicit: Implicit Association Test (IAT): https://implicit.harvard.edu/implicit/takeatest.html

REFERENCES

Ackerman-Barger, K., Boatright, D., Gonzalez-Colaso, R., Orozco, R. & Latimore, D. (2020). Seeking inclusion excellence: Understanding racial microaggressions as experienced by underrepresented medical and nursing students. *Academic Medicine, 95*(5), 758–763. https://doi.org/10.1097/ACM.0000000000003077

American Association of Colleges of Nursing. (2017). Diversity, equity, and inclusion in academic nursing. [Position statement]. https://www.aacnnursing.org/news-data/position-statements-white-papers/diversity-equity-and-inclusion-in-academic-nursing

Baker, R., Dee, T., Evans, B., & John, J. (2022). Bias in online classes: Evidence from a field experiment. *Economics of Education Review, 88*. https://doi.org/10.1016/j.econedurev.2022.102259

Benander, R., & Rankey, P. (2021). Designing and facilitating equitable and inclusive online courses. In R. Kumar & B. Refaei (Eds.), *Equity and inclusion in higher education: Strategies for teaching* (pp. 41–54). University of Cincinnati Press.

Brooks, R., & Grady, S. D. (2022). Course design considerations for inclusion and representation. [White paper]. Quality Matters. http://qualitymatters.org

Caruso Brown, A. E., Hobart, T. R., Botash, A. S., & Germain, L. J. (2019). Can a checklist ameliorate implicit bias in medical education? *Medical Education, 53*(5), 510 https://doi.org/10.1111/medu.13840

Crutchfield, J., Fisher, A. K., & Plummer, S. (2022). Best practices for antiracist education in virtual settings. *Advances in Social Work, 22*(2), 741–757. https://doi.org/10.18060/24962

Fruh, S., Taylor, S., Graves, R., Hayes, K., McDermott, R., Hauff, C., Williams, S., Sittig, S., Campbell, M., Hudson, G., Hall, H., Melnyk, B., & Barinas, J. (2021). Relationships among hope, body satisfaction, wellness habits, and stress in nursing students. *Journal of Professional Nursing, 37*(3), 640–647. https://doi.org/10.1016/j.profnurs.2021.01.009

He, F. X., Turnbull, B., Kirshbaum, M. N., Phillips, B., & Klainin-Yobas, P. (2018). Assessing stress, protective factors and psychological well-being among undergraduate nursing students. *Nurse Education Today, 68*, 4–12. https://doi.org/10.1016/j.nedt.2018.05.013

Iheduru-Anderson, K. C., & Wahi, M. M. (2021). Rejecting the myth of equal opportunity: An agenda to eliminate racism in nursing education in the United States. *BMC Nursing, 20*(1), 1–10. https://doi.org/10.1186/s12912-021-00548-9

Jennings, S., Mikos, K., Caruso Brown, A., Osborne, K., & Livesay, S. (2024). Evaluation of nursing coursework for biased content. *Nursing Education Perspectives, 45* (1), 53–54. https://doi.org/10.1097/01.NEP.0000000000001082

Kumar, R., & Refaei, B. (2021). *Equity and inclusion in higher education: Strategies for teaching.* University of Cincinnati Press.

Lee, C. N., & Hopson, M. (2019). Disrupting postracial discourse: Black millennials' response to postracial ideology and the continued impact of racial microaggressions on college campuses. *Southern Communication Journal, 84*(2), 127–139. https://doi.org/10.1080/1041794X.2018.1517186

Lin, P. S. L., & Kennette, L. N. (2021). Creating an inclusive learning community to better serve minority students. *Journal of Effective Teaching in Higher Education, 4*(3), 1–18. https://doi.org/10.36021/jethe.v4i3.250

Melendez, K., & Thompson, A. (2020). Cultural competency: A call to action to address microaggression in preservice health education. *Health Education Journal, 79*(7), 851–859. https://doi.org/10.1177/17896920921501

Miles, M., Brockman, A., & Naphan-Kingery, D. (2020). Invalidated identities: The disconfirming effects of racial microaggressions on Black doctoral students in STEM. *Journal of Research in Science Teaching, 57*, 1608–1631.

Miller, R. A., Howell, C. D., Oyarzun, B., Martin, F., Knight, S., & Frankovich, J. (2023). Faculty perspectives on inclusion, diversity, equity, and access (IDEA) in Online Teaching. *Online Learning, 27*(3), 387–406. https://doi.org/10.24059/olj.v27i3.3691

National Academies of Sciences, Engineering, and Medicine. (2021). *The future of nursing 2020–2030: Charting a path to achieve health equity.* National Academies Press. https://doi.org/10.17226/25982

National Center for Education Statistics. (2021). *Figure 2. Undergraduate enrollment in degree-granting postsecondary institutions, by race/ethnicity and nonresident status: Fall 2010, 2019, and 2021.* [Fast Facts]. https://nces.ed.gov/fastfacts/display.asp?id=98

The National Education Association. (2024). *Recognizing your biases.* https://www.nea.org/recognizing-your-biases

Pusey-Reid, E., Gona, C., Lussier-Duynstee, P., & Gall, G. (2022). Microaggressions: Microaggressions: Black students' experiences—a qualitative study. *Journal of Professional Nursing, 40*, 73–78. https://doi.org/10.1016/j.profnurs.2022.03.004

Sue, D. W. (2010). *Microaggressions in everyday life: Race, gender & sexual orientation*. John Wiley & Sons.

Sue, D. W., & Spanierman, L.B. (2020). *Microaggressions in everyday life.* (2nd ed.). John Wiley & Sons.

Sullivan, L. W. (2004). *Missing persons: Minorities in the health professions. A report of the Sullivan Commission on diversity in the healthcare workforce. https://campaignforaction.org/wp-content/uploads/2016/04/SullivanReport-Diversity-in-Healthcare-Workforce1.pdf*

Taylor, B., Zamaripa, C., Stevens, J., & Satre, M. (2023). Belonging in online nursing education. *Online Journal of Issues in Nursing, 28*(2). https://doi-org/10.3912/ojin.vol28no02man05

Zajac, L. (2015). The culture care meaning of comfort for ethnically diverse nursing students in the educational Setting. *Online Journal of Cultural Competence in Nursing and Healthcare, 5*(1), 88–103. http://dx.doi.org/10.9730/ojccnh.org/v5n1a7

Zajac, L., & Benton-Lee. J. (2023). Microaggressions: Experiences of diverse graduate nursing students in online education. *Journal of Transcultural Nursing, 34*(4), 301–309. https://doi.org/10.1177/10436596231166043

Zajac, L., & Lane, A. (2020). Student perceptions of faculty caring and social presence in online courses. *Quarterly Review of Distance Education, 21*(2), 67–78.

Zhuang-Shuang, L., & Hasson, F. (2020). Resilience, stress, and psychological well-being in nursing students: A systematic review. *Nurse Education Today, 90*. https://doi.org/10.1016/j.nedt.2020.104440

Credits

IMG 7.1: Source: https://nappy.co/photo/2383.

Icon 7.1: Apple icon is Copyright © by Microsoft.

Icon 7.2: Owl icon is Copyright © by Microsoft.

Icon 7.3: Slate icon is Copyright © by Microsoft.

Icon 7.4: Pencil icon is Copyright © by Microsoft.

Icon 7.5: Computer icon is Copyright © by Microsoft.

Appendix: Upstate Bias Checklist

A Checklist for Assessing Bias in Health Professions Education Content

Please reference the Upstate Bias Checklist Manual (https://implicit.harvard.edu/implicit/takeatest.html) for more information.

CURRICULUM

1. Curricular Unit
2. Course
3. TLM Title
4. TLM Type

RACE AND ETHNICITY

1. Does the content include any mention of race or ethnicity? If photos of humans or parts of humans are included, race is present in the content.
    - Yes
    - No
2. Should the content include any mention of race or ethnicity?
    - Yes
    - Unsure
    - No
3. Are explicit biological differences between racial or ethnic groups stated?
    - Yes
    - No
4. Regarding content about EXPLICIT biological differences between racial or ethnic groups, check all that apply:
    - This content is not essential to the lecture.
    - This content is not scientifically accurate.

- The relationship of social or structural determinants of health to the racial or ethnic differences is not discussed.
- This content does not discuss the role of toxic stress (e.g., chronic exposure to racism) in contributing to biological differences between races.
- This content states that racial groups are biological constructs.
- Learners are told that this information is important for standardized examinations.
- None of the above applies to this content.

5. Are biological differences between racial or ethnic groups implied?

   - Yes
   - No

6. Regarding content about IMPLICIT biological differences between racial or ethnic groups, check all that apply:

   - This content is not essential to the lecture.
   - This content is not scientifically accurate.
   - The relationship of social or structural determinants of health to the racial or ethnic differences is not discussed.
   - This content does not discuss the role of toxic stress (e.g., chronic exposure to racism) in contributing to biological differences between races.
   - This content implies that racial groups are biological constructs.
   - Learners are told that this information is important for standardized examinations.
   - None of the above applies to this content.

7. Could this content be perceived as promoting stereotypes, bias, shame, or stigma?

   - Yes
   - Unsure
   - No

Recommendations

VISUAL IMAGES

1. Were visual images of human beings included?
   - Yes
   - No
2. Was consent obtained for use of these images?
   - Yes
   - No
3. Do the images add something important to the content?
   - Yes
   - No
4. Could the image(s) suggest stereotypes or promote bias?
   Be particularly cautious with cartoons and other images that are meant to be comical, as well as with images that are de-identified in some way (headless, eyes covered with black bars-these may imply that the person photographed should be ashamed of being identified and the latter are ineffective).
   - Yes
   - Unsure
   - No

5. Are the people depicted in the images racially and ethnically diverse?
   - Yes
   - No
6. Are the people depicted in the images diverse in terms of body habitus (e.g., shape, size, physical disability)?
   - Yes
   - No
7. If using images of physical findings, do they represent the full spectrum of skin tones or other physical features?
   - Yes
   - No
   - Not Applicable
8. If using image(s) to illustrate morphological features of disability, are the image(s) primarily tragic or negative (e.g., suggesting a poor quality of life)?
   - Yes
   - Unsure
   - No

Recommendations

CLINICAL VIGNETTES

1. Does your content contain one or more clinical vignettes or references to specific patients (whether real or hypothetical)?
   - Yes
   - No
2. Are patients' stories de-identified or was consent obtained for the use of their stories in teaching?
   - De-identified
   - Verbal or written consent obtained
   - Both de-identified and consent obtained
   - Neither de-identified nor consent obtained
   - Patient cases are all hypothetical
3. Does the vignette use language that indicates judgment of the patient or the patient's behavior?
   In addition to more obvious examples, subtle word choices (such as "alleged", "admitted" or "denied") may also indicate judgment and should be avoided in most cases.
   - Yes
   - Unsure
   - No
4. Is any aspect of the (real or hypothetical) patient's experience mocked, shamed, or demeaned?
   Includes any comments meant to elicit laughter, sarcasm, etc.
   - Yes
   - Unsure
   - No

Recommendations

SEX AND GENDER

1. Does the content include any mention of sex or gender?
   If photos of humans are included or if the content includes clinical vignettes/references to individual people (patients or health care professionals), gender is most likely present in the content.
   - Yes
   - No
2. Should the content include any mention of sex or gender?
   - Yes
   - Unsure
   - No
3. Are all genders represented in the content?
   - Yes
   - Unsure
   - No
4. Is gender presented as part of a spectrum (i.e., NOT represented as a binary concept)?
   - Yes
   - No

5. Does the content conflate gender identity with sexual orientation?
   - Yes
   - Unsure
   - No
6. Does the content promote traditional gender roles?
   - Yes
   - Unsure
   - No
7. Are symptoms, signs, other clinical findings and/or disease presentations (e.g., chest pain) referred to as "atypical" or "variant" when they occur in women?
   - Yes
   - No
8. Could the content be perceived as promoting stereotypes, bias, shame, or stigma?
   - Yes
   - Unsure
   - No

Recommendations

SEXUALITY, SEXUAL BEHAVIOR, AND SEXUAL ORIENTATION

1. Does the content include any mention of sexual behavior, sexuality, or sexual orientation?
   - Yes
   - No
2. Should the content include any mention of sexual behavior, sexuality, or sexual orientation?
   - Yes
   - Unsure
   - No
3. Is the spectrum of sexual orientation represented in the content?
   - Yes
   - Unsure
   - No
4. Does the content recognize the sexual health needs of patients with physical disabilities?
   - Yes
   - Unsure
   - No
5. Does the content recognize the sexual health needs of patients with cognitive disabilities?
   - Yes
   - Unsure
   - No
6. Does the content recognize the sexual health needs of older patients, including geriatric patients?
   - Yes
   - Unsure
   - No

7. Could the content be perceived as promoting stereotypes, bias, shame, or stigma?
   - Yes
   - Unsure
   - No

Recommendations

DISABILITY

1. Does the content include any mention of disability, including physical or cognitive/intellectual disability? *Note that mental health, substance use, and aging are addressed in separate domains.*
   - Yes
   - No
2. Should the content include any mention of disability, including physical or cognitive/intellectual disability?
   - Yes
   - Unsure
   - No
3. Does the content include positive representations of disability (e.g., as typical human variation or diversity)?
   - Yes
   - Unsure
   - No

4. Could the content be perceived as promoting stereotypes, bias, shame, or stigma?
   - Yes
   - Unsure
   - No

Recommendations

MENTAL HEALTH AND SUBSTANCE USE

1. Does the content include any mention of mental health or substance use?
   - Yes
   - No
2. Should the content include any mention of mental health or substance use, or of the particular healthcare needs of patients with these concerns?
   - Yes
   - Unsure
   - No

3. Could the content be perceived as promoting stereotypes, bias, shame, or stigma?

   - Yes
   - Unsure
   - No

Recommendations

WEIGHT

1. Does the content include any mention of weight or body mass index?

   - Yes
   - No

2. Does the content assume or imply a linear or straightforward relationship between weight (or body mass index) and health?

   - Yes
   - Unsure
   - No

3. Does the content emphasize personal responsibility in discussions of obesity?

   - Yes
   - Unsure
   - No

4. Does the content discuss genetic, epigenetic, social, and structural risk factors related to obesity?
   - Yes
   - Unsure
   - No
5. Could the content be perceived as promoting stereotypes, bias, shame, or stigma?
   - Yes
   - Unsure
   - No

Recommendations

IMMIGRATION STATUS, NATIONALITY, LANGUAGE, AND CULTURE

1. Does the content include any mention of immigration status, nationality, language, or culture?
   - Yes
   - No
2. Should this content include any discussion of the healthcare needs of patients who are not citizens, were born in another country, or do not speak English fluently?
   - Yes
   - Unsure
   - No

3. Does this content distinguish between different categories of immigration status, including refugees, asylum seekers, and undocumented immigrants, "green card holders", etc.?
   - Yes
   - No
   - Not applicable
4. Could this content be understood as suggesting that patients who do not speak English are less capable of understanding healthcare information, making informed healthcare decisions or adhering to healthcare recommendations?
   - Yes
   - Unsure
   - No
5. Could the content be perceived as promoting stereotypes, bias, shame, or stigma?
   - Yes
   - Unsure
   - No

Recommendations

POVERTY AND SOCIOECONOMIC STATUS

1. Does the content include any mention of poverty or socioeconomic status?
   - Yes
   - No
2. Should this content include a discussion of poverty or socioeconomic status?
   - Yes
   - Unsure
   - No
3. Could the content be perceived as promoting stereotypes, bias, shame, or stigma?
   - Yes
   - Unsure
   - No

Recommendations

AGE

1. Does the content include any discussion of older adults or geriatric patients?

   - Yes
   - No

2. Should this content include a discussion of the distinctive needs of older adults or geriatric patients?
   Considerations include whether the issue being taught often affects older people or manifests differently in older people. Pay special attention to discussions of sexuality.

   - Yes
   - Unsure
   - No

3. Could the content be perceived as promoting stereotypes, bias, shame, or stigma?

   - Yes
   - Unsure
   - No

Recommendations

RELIGION AND FAITH TRADITION

1. Does the content include any discussion of religion or faith tradition?
   - Yes
   - No
2. Should this content include any discussion of religion or of the special needs of patients belonging to certain religious groups or faith traditions?
   Please use caution in this area and avoid treating religious groups as monolithic; most patients interpret their religious faith or lack thereof in ways unique to them and their families.
   - Yes
   - Unsure
   - No
3. Does that content assume that religious or faith-based groups are monolithic and present their beliefs as such?
   Examples include suggesting that all Muslim women refuse to see male providers; that all Amish families want to consult their community elders prior to making a major medical decision; or that Catholic patients never use contraception.
   - Yes
   - Unsure
   - No
4. Could the content be perceived as promoting stereotypes, bias, shame, or stigma?
   - Yes
   - Unsure
   - No

Recommendations

PRISONERS

1. Does the content include any discussion of incarceration or of the special healthcare needs of prisoners?
   - Yes
   - No
2. Should this content include any discussion of incarceration or of the special healthcare needs of prisoners?
   - Yes
   - Unsure
   - No
3. Does the content discuss mass incarceration as a public health problem (e.g., the school-to-prison pipeline)?
   - Yes
   - No
4. Does the content discuss the relationship between systemic, institutional, or structural racism and mass incarceration?
   - Yes
   - No

5. Could the content be perceived as promoting stereotypes, bias, shame, or stigma?
   - Yes
   - Unsure
   - No

Recommendations

RURAL RESIDENCE

1. Does this content include any discussion of patients from or of healthcare provision in rural areas?
   - Yes
   - No
2. Should this content include any discussion of the particular healthcare needs of rural patients and populations?
   - Yes
   - Unsure
   - No
3. Could the content be perceived as promoting stereotypes, bias, shame, or stigma?
   - Yes
   - Unsure
   - No

Recommendations

INTERPROFESSIONAL COMMUNICATION

1. Does this content discuss healthcare practitioners from more than one profession (e.g., medicine, nursing, physical therapy) or specialty (e.g., pediatrics, emergency medicine)?
   - Yes
   - No
2. Should this content discuss healthcare practitioners from more than one profession (e.g., medicine, nursing, physical therapy) or specialty (e.g., pediatrics, emergency medicine)?
   - Yes
   - Unsure
   - No
3. Does this content address each profession and/or specialty respectfully?
   - Yes
   - Unsure
   - No
4. Does this content use gender-neutral pronouns when referring to members of each profession or specialty?
   - Yes
   - Unsure
   - No

5. Could the content be perceived as promoting stereotypes, bias, shame, or stigma?
    - Yes
    - Unsure
    - No

Recommendations

FINAL COMMENTS AND RECOMMENDATIONS

CHAPTER 8

Caring, Communication, and Social Presence

Teaching Online for Virtual and Telehealth Nursing Roles

"Unless we are making progress in our nursing every year, every month, every week, take my word for it, we are going back."

—FLORENCE NIGHTINGALE

TERMS TO KNOW

telecare: Refers to the technology that consumers use to improve health and wellness. Select examples include apps for tracking exercise and nutrition, and sensors and tools for monitoring blood glucose, cardiac arrhythmias, detecting falls and other health conditions.

telehealth: A means of providing health care through electronic communication and technology where the healthcare professional and the patient are separated by distance. Telehealth is a broad term that also encompasses clinical health care, patient and professional health-related education, public health, and health administration. In this chapter, telehealth refers to an e-health visit with the primary healthcare provider through electronic means. Examples of professionals who provide care via telehealth are nurses, pharmacists, social workers, speech therapists, audiologists, physical therapists, and physicians.

telemedicine: Provision of medical care or medicine, usually between a physician and patient, by electronic means. Sometimes used interchangeably with *telehealth*.

telepresence: A set of behaviors that can be used to describe a positive experience in a telehealth visit.

virtual integrated care (VIC): Virtual nursing; the virtual nurse is incorporated as a member of the healthcare team and establishes a visible online presence through the teleconference camera in the hospital room to observe and examine the patient.

virtual nursing: A nursing care delivery mode where nurses work remotely via computer through videoconferencing to care for patients through observation and communication and by performing nursing actions that require presence but not physical proximity. Select examples of care actions include conducting admission interviews, providing patient teaching, and giving discharge instructions.

virtual social presence: The process of exhibiting oneself as human in the online environment by expressing emotion and displaying social actions.

Chapter Overview and Objectives

Online nurse educators teach a variety of students, including those who graduate and become advanced practice nurses and virtual nurses. Online caring actions and presence are important skills for these roles. This chapter provides the learner with information about virtual nursing and telehealth, including definitions, challenges, and successes associated with the hospital virtual nurse and advanced practice registered nurse practitioner using telehealth. Essential caring skills, positive presence behaviors, therapeutic communication, and netiquette associated with virtual nursing situations are presented. Current research and interviews that demonstrate the healthcare providers' lived experiences associated with virtual nursing and telehealth are explored. Opportunities for learners to discuss and role model appropriate caring actions in virtual nursing situations are provided.

In this chapter, the learner will:

1. Define *virtual nursing* and *telehealth* as influenced by technology and healthcare expansion.
2. Compare and contrast the barriers to and benefits of virtual nursing and telehealth related to online caring and communication.
3. Discuss appropriate communication skills for exhibiting caring and telepresence in telehealth and virtual nursing.
4. Determine components of telehealth and virtual nursing content associated with caring, empathy, and online presence for nursing education.
5. Develop a plan for modeling caring, empathy, and telehealth netiquette behaviors for use during telehealth nursing visits and virtual nurse activities.

Virtual Nursing and Telehealth: Online Nursing Practice

If you are a nurse educator and teaching online, chances are you will have nurse educator students who will someday teach nurses who are or will be virtual nurses in the hospital setting or advanced practice registered nurses (APRNs) using telehealth. Chapter 6 covers the art of virtual caring and social presence in nursing education from a nurse-educator perspective. This chapter supports online education about caring, presence, compassion, and immediacy as vital skills for the telehealth and virtual nursing milieu.

Nursing is a profession known for caring, compassion, competence, and application of scientific principles in the health care of people. The American Nurses Association (ANA) states that

> Nursing integrates the art and science of caring and focuses on the protection, promotion, and optimization of health and human functioning; prevention of illness and injury; facilitation of healing; and alleviation of suffering through compassionate presence. Nursing is the diagnosis and treatment of human responses and advocacy in the care of individuals, families,

> groups, communities, and populations in recognition of the connection of all humanity. (2021, para. 1)

A key phrase of the ANA definition of nursing is *compassionate presence.* Compassionate presence should not be dependent upon physical location. Newer methods of nursing care and advanced practice nursing have evolved over the past several years and include the concept of virtual nursing and telehealth; the nursing care is provided remotely so that the patient is in one location and the registered nurse or advanced practice nurse is in another. Carroll discusses nurses' opportunities for telehealth from the position of the art of nursing through the use of Parse's theory of human becoming; telehealth is the means by which the care is delivered, but it is the nurse who provides presence, guided by the human becoming theory of Rosemarie Parse, to understand the meaning of the patient's experience, values, and interactions in the context of health (Carroll, 2018).

Introduction to Virtual Nursing

Virtual nursing has emerged due to the current and projected shortage of registered nurses (Health Resources and Services Administration [HRSA], 2022). By 2036, projections are that the United States will be short 337,970 full-time RNs (Bean, 2024). Virtual nursing is one answer to the projected nursing shortage as it decreases the number of nurses needed and is designed to minimize workload and stress, which are two significant reasons for nurses leaving the profession (Auerbach et al., 2022). Virtual nursing, or virtual integrated care, is a healthcare delivery mode where nurses work remotely via computer and videoconferencing to care for patients through observation and communication and by performing nursing actions that require presence but not physical proximity. Hospital patient rooms are either pre-equipped for videoconferencing with the computer screen present in the room, or the computer screen is attached to a pole and wheeled into the patient's room when the virtual nurse is part of the care team. Select examples of nursing care actions include conducting admission interviews, providing patient teaching, giving discharge instructions, verifying medication, engaging in decision-making, and monitoring patients, which frees up the bedside nurse for hands-on care and other actions requiring physical presence.

Virtual Nursing Care Delivery Models

Various models of virtual nursing care delivery have been developed, and the model used in a healthcare facility often depends on the available resources and the location facility; for example, rural hospitals may have different staffing needs when compared to metropolitan hospitals. A major goal of virtual nursing is to improve the workload of the bedside nurse without higher costs or compromising patient care. Several models of virtual nursing care delivery aim to accomplish this. One example is a model where the hospital hires a nurse for the virtual nurse position or hires a nurse from an employment agency to fill the virtual nurse role. The virtual nurse is located at a communication or command center within the hospital and is able to support several bedside nurses at one time. Or the hospital hires the virtual nurse for this position to work remotely from home. Another model uses a hybrid approach where nurses share the bedside and virtual nurse roles. For example, each week a nurse may work two shifts at the bedside and one shift as the virtual nurse. The hybrid model is associated with trust and collaboration among nurses and high nurse satisfaction (Loughlin, 2023). Another model uses a team approach, which comprises a virtual nurse, a bedside registered nurse, and a licensed practical nurse (Poirier, 2023) who provide care to a group of patients. Additional models include the use of the virtual nurse as a sitter or observer for patients who are high risk for falls and the use of experienced virtual nurses to support new nurses on a unit (Delaney, 2022; Poirier, 2023).

Benefits of Virtual Nursing

Virtual nursing is designed for continuous care during a patient's hospital stay. Telehealth or telemedicine, which is episodic, offers other benefits discussed later in the chapter. Virtual nursing is not new; in fact, tele-ICUs have existed since 1977 (Vranas et al., 2018). Different ways to utilize the virtual nursing model grew during the COVID-19 pandemic, as evidenced by the plethora of literature available on the topic since 2019. Research is ongoing; however, preliminary reports reveal that patient satisfaction, safety, and infection rates are improved with the use of virtual nursing (Sanford et al., 2023). More research is needed in all areas to determine continued benefits and improved outcomes with virtual nursing care delivery models (National Council of State Boards of Nursing [NCSBN],

2024). The cost of virtual nursing continues to be an issue as hospitals look for a positive return on the investment (Wicklund, 2023).

Other benefits are that nurses who are retired or close to retirement and still desire to share their expertise but cannot meet the physical demands of bedside nursing may choose to work remotely from home as a virtual nurse (HCA Healthcare, 2024). Nurses with physical disabilities can also work virtually/remotely for similar reasons. Patients enjoy knowing that there is someone to look in on them and who is available to promptly answer their questions; subsequently, patient satisfaction scores are on the increase (Sanford et al., 2023; Wicklund, 2023), as is perceived nurse satisfaction with the experience (HCA Healthcare, 2024).

Challenges to Virtual Nursing

Barriers to virtual nursing include costs and sustainability, concerns about quality of care, equipment and technology issues, and organizational leadership impatience with waiting on results of the cost-benefit of the programs; a consequence of unresolved challenges may be the discontinuation of programs (Wicklund, 2023). Other explanations for failed virtual nursing programs include delays in program implementation, lack of collaboration between the beside nurse and the virtual nurse, communication issues, and lack of or inappropriate technology (Loughlin, 2023).

The key to a successful virtual nurse program is adequate planning and having the right people at the decision-making table (Loughlin, 2023). See Box 8.1 for resources and steps needed for successful implementation of virtual nursing in a healthcare facility.

Healthcare facilities need to determine what works best for a virtual nursing care model in the organization. Read *Experiences from the Virtual Field* in Box 8.2 for an interview between nurse informaticist Dr. CJ Wachs, DNP, RN (director of informatics at a level 1 trauma center in the Midwest) and the book author about the use of virtual nursing models and the importance of presence, trust, and caring with these models, as well as how to prepare nursing students for the virtual nursing setting.

Dr. Wachs presented thoughts and recommendations about virtual nursing and telehealth from a nurse informaticist's perspective. The ideas represent a commitment to patient care and caring communication between nurses and from nurses to patients.

BOX 8.1 Resources Needed to Plan and Implement a Hospital Virtual Nurse Program

1. An interprofessional planning/implementation team: Team should include the chief financial officer (CFO), HR representative, chief nursing officer (CNO), virtual nurse champions, staff nurses, nurse informaticist, IT representative, hardware engineer, infection-control healthcare provider, QI person, and end users, which could include a patient representative.
2. Healthcare facility: Consider the pros and cons of old versus new.
3. Delivery care model: Decide on format.
4. Virtual nurse location: Decide on home or in a designated room at the healthcare facility.
5. Financial resources: Determine the return on investment (ROI):
   a. Startup technology costs
   b. Implementation: Technology, orientation of the team
   c. Salary of agency versus staff nurses
   d. Cost savings of using virtual nurse
5. Technological capability: Bandwidth, promptness of repairs, ability to sustain the virtual nurse program.
6. Virtual nurses: Consider candidates with strong communication skills for virtual/online patient and healthcare team interactions.
7. Communication skills: Interactions between the bedside nurses and virtual nurses.
   a. Trust
   b. Collaboration
   c. Video screen training: Online caring, presence, and compassion/empathy
   d. Workflows between the bedside nurse and virtual nurse

Adapted from: Delaney, M. (2022, September 1). Patient-centered care: The rise of the virtual nurse. *HealthTech.* https://healthtechmagazine.net/article/2022/09/rise-virtual-nurse; Loughlin, B. (2023, July 18). Virtual nursing: The radical transformation of the way nurses work. [Webinar]. American Nursing Informatics Association. https://library.ania.org/conferences/1/view; Sanford, K., Schuelke, S., Lee, M., & Mossburg, S. E. (2023, August 30). *Virtual nursing: Improving patient care and meeting workforce challenges.* PSNet. https://psnet.ahrq.gov/perspective/virtual-nursing-improving-patient-care-and-meeting-workforce-challenges

BOX 8.2 Experience from the Virtual Field: Interview on Virtual Nursing and Caring

Question: How would you describe your experience with virtual nursing?

Dr. Wachs: I have held several positions of nursing leadership around virtual nursing. First, I was a staff nurse in the hospital to gain experience, followed by the role of nurse informaticist to help nurses in the area of informatics and technology. As a nurse informaticist, I supported nurses who used telehealth when it was in its infancy. My doctoral project focused on how to use technology in a novel way to support nurses and nursing care. I created a new model of nursing, collaborating with other disciplines.

Question: What are your perceptions about the benefits of virtual nursing?

Dr. Wachs: One benefit is that nurses have the opportunity to work from home. I support the hybrid virtual nurse care delivery method where a nurse can work on the unit 1 or 2 days per week; in addition, the same nurse can work from home as a virtual nurse for the same nursing unit—paired with a face-to-face nurse 1 to 2 days per week. This is part of the solution to staff nursing burnout and the nursing shortage. Another benefit is that the use of the virtual nurse model is a way for hospitals to retain aging nurses because the virtual nursing work is less physical for them while keeping the older nurses' expertise and experience. Virtual nurses can also help with the precepting and mentoring of novice nurses.

Question: What are your perceptions about the challenges or barriers with virtual nursing?

Dr. Wachs: Trust is an issue for the traditional approach to virtual nursing where the virtual nurses stay virtual and the bedside nurses stay at the bedside. In other words, nurses working in person don't trust the virtual nurse and vice versa. If these nurses aren't familiar with each other there could be trust issues about the care and knowledge each brings to the table. A way to resolve this is the hybrid approach, which I discussed previously, using the nurse pairs who move back and forth between the virtual nurse and the in-patient nurse role. Virtual nursing is not a one-size-fits-all approach—need to use a model that is best for the organization. Another issue is that virtual nurses need to learn about how to advise other nurses as well as care for patients through the use of a computer.

Question: How do you convey caring in a virtual educational or practice setting?

Dr. Wachs: Caring is the heart of nursing. Interaction matters! One can't just be transactional; the nurse needs to be interactive and transformative. Virtual nurses are called on to determine ways to stay connected to the nurses they are working with and the patients they are caring for. I do wonder about a communication skill set for virtual nurses and have questions. Can caring be learned? Should there be a minimal competency for communication and caring connection?

Question: Where do you see virtual nursing in the future?

Dr. Wachs: I see more healthcare facilities moving to telehealth and the use of the hospital-at-home model, which relies on telehealth and virtual nursing. Hospitals need to consider the return on investment when determining the use of virtual nursing for this model.

Question: What should students know about virtual nursing?

Dr. Wachs: At the undergraduate level, nursing students need to learn therapeutic communication and assessment competencies well, and students need actual clinical experience to use these basic competencies before adding a virtual component. Then, the students can practice or simulate virtual nursing with each other. Practicing with the technology removes some of the barriers to using the virtual nursing model when the student enters nursing practice. Also, undergraduate students can learn about issues related to privacy/HIPAA with telehealth and virtual nursing.

At the graduate level, nursing informatics courses should contain information about virtual nursing and telehealth, including how to do assessments and use therapeutic communication in a virtual setting.

Introduction to Telehealth

Telehealth is a means of providing health care through technology, specifically electronic communication, where the healthcare professional and the patient are separated by distance. Examples of professionals who engage in telehealth are nurses, pharmacists, and social workers. Care is usually episodic, representing one patient and healthcare professional/provider encounter using common technology such as computers, smartphones, tablets, videoconference software, and internet connections. The terms *telehealth* and *telemedicine* are often used similarly; however, *telehealth* has a wider range and requires a sender and a receiver (Health.IT.gov, 2019) For more information on terms, see ONC https://www.healthit.gov/faq/why-telehealth-important-rural-providers located under Chapter Resources.

Benefits to Telehealth

Telehealth originated in the 1950s with use of closed-circuit TV for medical consultations and then slowly expanded over the decades as technology developed with the growth of the internet and digital communication and use of the electronic health records (EHR); telehealth became mainstream by the first decade of the millennium (Board on Health Care Services, Institute of Medicine, 2012; Garber et al., 2023). Telehealth use for patient care increased during the COVID-19 pandemic, and telehealth provider visits continue to increase (Rettinger & Kuhn, 2023).

Patients like the widespread use of telehealth and express satisfaction with telehealth care because of increased access to quality care and services, lack of travel, and ability to stay at home (Gajarawala & Pelkowski, 2021). Additional benefits include lower provider and patient costs, less onsite healthcare, provider satisfaction with the telehealth modality, and improved patient outcomes, especially in rural areas (Butzner & Cuffee, 2021).

Challenges in Telehealth

Challenges related to the use of videoconferencing for telehealth provider visits include issues associated with technology; practice issues, such as lack of hands-on care; administrative issues; patient and environmental issues; and interpersonal/communication issues (Rettinger & Kuhn, 2023).

Additional barriers and challenges to telehealth usage include technology issues such as lack of adequate internet connection in rural or underserved areas, legal issues associated with e-visits across state lines, privacy issues with the use of electronic devices for the telehealth encounter, provider e-visit regulations, and medical liability issues related to the electronic modalities and patient care (Gajarawala & Pelkowski, 2021). Communication issues and lack of knowledge contribute to the telehealth challenge; the increase in telehealth as a modality for patient visits prompts the development of learning modules and curricular additions to advanced practice nursing education and professional health programs (Browne et al., 2022; Chike-Harris et al., 2021; Herrera & Foronda, 2022).

Ashely Harris, MSN, FNP-BC, APRN, is an experienced telehealth nurse and leader at a home healthcare call center. She manages and conducts telehealth visits and completes virtual assessments while paired with a registered nurse who is at the patient's home. Ms. Harris responded to questions during an interview with the book author about her experiences with telehealth and virtual caring using this paired model. See Box 8.3.

BOX 8.3 Experience from the Virtual Field: Interview About Telehealth and Caring

Question: Describe your experience with virtual nursing and telehealth.

Ms. Harris: I work with older adults who usually have Medicare insurance. These patients tend to be less tech-savvy. I communicate with the patients for telehealth visits either via computer or phone; the majority of the telehealth visits are by phone. The goal of the healthcare company that I work for is to prevent unnecessary hospitalizations; so, we offer telehealth services 24/7. Telehealth call topics range from patients asking health questions, or wanting to know if they should go to the hospital, and/or assessments for urgent care.

Question: What are your perceptions of the benefits of virtual nursing/telehealth?

Ms. Harris: Telehealth reaches people who wouldn't otherwise have access to health care and/or keeps patients from getting lost in the system; some older adults have anxiety about technology, so I use the phone for calls, which is a form of telehealth. Other benefits are that I can talk to families about caregiver strain, I can educate patients about their health, and then, if needed, I send in an RN to the home. Advanced practice nurses are available for telehealth during the week, the weekend, and after hours. Personally, the telehealth setting worked for me during COVID; I did not want to risk being sick with a daughter at home. Because of the telehealth setup, I can spend more time at my home with [my] daughter. Professionally, there are opportunities for growth and leadership in the company and opportunities for creativity with the evolving telehealth role.

Question: What are your perceptions of the challenges or barriers?

Ms. Harris: From the nursing side—transitioning from face-to-face to the phone or video is challenging; one has to be clinically sound and be aware what you know or don't know. Currently, there is no standardization yet for telehealth care. Distraction while on the phone can be an issue. The telehealth advance practice nurse has to have good listening skills and be able to think critically through situations as described on the phone by the patient. Also, technology disruptions could be a challenge. I may have to talk a patient through the technology of a telehealth visit or talk with a family member who is present to help. Health privacy can be an issue for a patient at home. The telehealth APRN makes sure that phone visits are OK with the patient if family members are present.

Question: How do you convey caring in a virtual practice setting?

Ms. Harris: The visit is what you make it. There should be no difference in caring during an in-person visit versus the phone visit. I don't always see a face—I really listen; I allow space/time for the patient to talk; I listen for voice changes in the patient; I smile when I talk so I remain positive in my conversation. I do have conversation prompts which are helpful. I also end the conversation with "I am or we are available."

In a video telehealth situation, which uses more natural interaction because of the face-to-face encounter, the patients can see my smile. Whether it's a phone or video visit, I treat the caller like they are my grandmother, which helps me connect with them. I always find something to connect to them.

With either format, I try to make sure the technology of telehealth is not disruptive to the visit. My actions should match my words and tone of voice whether I am teaching or ending the visit. This is how caring occurs in virtual nursing.

Question: Where do you see virtual nursing/telehealth in the future?

Ms. Harris: I believe it will continue to grow.

Question: What should students know about virtual nursing?

Ms. Harris: For undergraduates, let undergraduates know that with therapeutic conversation, quiet moments are OK, remember "the pause," learn how to stop and redirect. Communication is vital to virtual nursing. Best practices are to introduce oneself, listen, watch tone of voice, allow for silence and also space for communication. Consider what they [the patient] are not saying and remember to incorporate the patient's family members when appropriate.

For graduate nursing students, it depends on what their role will be. Teaching should include education that targets communication as well as assessment in the virtual setting. In addition, education about how one makes good clinical decisions in the virtual setting would be appropriate. Engage graduate nursing students in research about best practices for telehealth.

Question: Any other ideas or comments?

Ms. Harris: You have to know how to be a nurse first and then make the transition to telehealth. Don't let the telehealth [technology] platform trip you up. Don't give up and consider the patient goals during the visit. I believe that tapping into the humanity of the person will allow you to be successful in telehealth.

Online Caring Skills for the Virtual Nurse

The benefits and challenges of virtual nursing for continuous hospital care and telehealth for episodic visits demonstrate the need for the development of policies, standardization of care, workforce regulation and planning, and expansion of nursing education and continuing education (Rambur et al., 2019); "new and renewed skills are needed to provide safe, effective, culturally relevant telehealth, and virtual care" (p. 64). Furthermore, Sanford et al. (2023) call on healthcare organizations to advance virtual care technology and hire nurses capable in the virtual role who have effective communication abilities.

Teaching Caring Communication for Telehealth and Virtual Nursing

Currently, there is no standardization of practice for virtual nursing/telehealth; thus, the literature on incorporating virtual nursing/telehealth concepts into nursing curricula is limited. Teaching content about virtual nursing environments and providing practice opportunities should occur at all levels of nursing education. The need also exists to teach interpersonal skills for communication in the context of telehealth (Henry et al., 2017). Current literature is limited about specific communication actions or behaviors for interactions in the telehealth/virtual environment. Caring actions and strong communication skills specific to the virtual healthcare environment, along with telehealth etiquette and best practices (Herrera & Foronda, 2022; Pravecek et al., 2024), are needed and should be included in nursing education programs. Faculty can focus on therapeutic communication skills and assessment competency at the undergraduate level and introduce virtual nursing as a nursing care delivery model. Education for advanced practice nursing students at the graduate level must include advanced assessment, observation, communication skills, and decision-making in the virtual setting as well. Love and Carrington (2021) created an educational project for advanced practice students that included seven modules covering content about:

1. Telehealth in practice and consultation
2. Rationale for telehealth for practice

3. Enhancement of consultation and collaboration with providers using telehealth
4. Privacy and confidentiality issues related to telehealth
5. Equipment utilized and common issues for telehealth
6. Ethical and legal implications of telehealth in practice
7. How to assess patient's willingness and knowledge to use required technology for telehealth

Each student engaged in a telehealth visit with a simulated patient; the visit was recorded for student debriefing, and the students and the simulated patients felt positive about the learning experience. Subsequently, the nursing program now offers a telehealth certificate that includes 90 hours of telehealth experience with a provider in addition to the modules and simulated experience (Love & Covington, 2021).

Online and face-to-face graduate students enrolled in advanced practice nursing programs and students who subsequently become virtual nurses will benefit from learning how to convey caring and compassion, social presence or telepresence, and immediacy behaviors in virtual practice environments. Students can learn to carry over therapeutic communication skills to the virtual environment, as noted in the example in Box 8.4. The skills listed can be applied to the virtual therapeutic nurse–patient interaction.

Caring Skills for Virtual Nurses

Thought leaders in business and health care offer virtual nursing as the answer to tech-driven, safe delivery of care and emphasize the importance of communication. For example, Scurlock (2023) states "virtual health care reinforces the idea that technology and compassion can seamlessly coexist, enriching the healthcare experience for all" (para. 11). However, there is minimal discussion in the literature specifically about what constitutes compassionate, caring, online communication in the virtual nursing practice setting and in telehealth. In addition to established standards of practice, virtual nurses and advanced practice nurses in telehealth should understand how to appear on camera and communicate with patients through technology, exhibiting telepresence, telehealth netiquette, and telehealth empathy (Wochcieckowski, 2023).

BOX 8.4 Select Therapeutic Communication Actions for the Virtual Nurse and APRN

Keys to Therapeutic Conversation

- Allow for pauses and quiet space.
- Listen for cues from the patient.
- Observe the patient's nonverbal actions.
- Avoid interrupting the patient.

Express empathy through validation of the patient's words and feelings.

- "It seems like you are feeling..."
- "You have been through a lot..."
- "I must be a lot of stress to handle..."
- "I respect your positive attitude..."
- "I am here to help..."
- "How are you coping..."

Adapted from: Hashim, M. J. (2017). Patient-centered communication: Basic skills. *American Family Physician*, *95*(1), 29–34.

Telepresence

Online or social presence is the process of exhibiting oneself as human in the online environment by expressing emotion and displaying social actions. *Telepresence* is a term that historically meant the presence of technology within a certain space. Barbosa-Angles and Hamilton (2020) expanded the term through qualitative study, identifying the characteristics that contribute to telepresence in a video telehealth visit: (1) body language, (2) eye contact, (3) verbal communication, (4) therapeutic relationship building, (5) acknowledging the presence of technology, and (7) patient and provider presentation on the screen.

Telehealth Netiquette

Garber et al. (2023) put forth a framework for telehealth based on the premise that netiquette is "not based on what care is delivered virtually, but how it is delivered virtually" (para. 8). The framework includes netiquette tips in three vital areas—performance, environment, and privacy/security—known as PEP (Garber et al., 2023). Table 8.1 describes each PEP component.

TABLE 8.1 PEP Framework for Telehealth Encounters with Essential Components

Element	Essentials
Performance	• Professional behavior ▪ Avoid eating/drinking during visits. • Use self-view to ensure screen position, "passport view." • Be punctual. • Confirm the patient can see/hear the provider at the start of the visit. • Communication ▪ Make eye contact. ▪ Begin with a confident introduction and identify your institution. ▪ Speak clearly and at a slower pace than normal. ▪ Consider lag time. • Wait 2–3 seconds to respond. ▪ Set agenda for the visit. • Identify patient priorities. • Summarize the plan for the visit. ▪ Use relationship-centered communication. • Be authentic and genuine. • Use nonverbal cues to project warmth, interest, and concern. • Deliberately nod, smile, and use facial expressions. • Engage with the patient to establish rapport. • Communicate empathy verbally and nonverbally. ▪ Employ a closing checklist. • Ensure the patient has an opportunity to ask questions. • Summarize the plan of care and post visit plan. • Provide clear follow-up instructions. • Provide a mechanism for the patient to contact the provider. • Technology proficiency ▪ Ensure provider knowledge of equipment and troubleshooting at both the provider and patient sites. • Establish skills to maximize the virtual exam, especially if using peripherals. • Keep technology support contact information readily available.

(Continued)

TABLE 8.1 (Continued)

Element	Essentials

Environment	• Personal appearance
	  ■ Dress professionally and/or wear a lab coat.
	  ■ Wear identification at eye level.
	  ■ Avoid active colors.
	  ■ Avoid distracting jewelry.
	• Provider setting
	  ■ Place light behind the camera, not the provider.
	  ■ Place webcam at eye level.
	  ■ Sit at a desk or table.
	  ■ Display professional items behind the provider, such as diplomas or institution name.
	  ■ Use a blue background when possible.
	• Avoid visual distractions.
	  ■ Remove clutter and inappropriate items from patient view.
	  ■ Avoid distracting objects/virtual backgrounds behind the provider.
	• Avoid auditory distractions.
	  ■ Type softly.
	  ■ Avoid television, music, or noise in background.
	  ■ Turn off cell phone and email alerts.
	  ■ Keep door closed during visits.
	• Technology
	  ■ Ensure strong connection via Wi-Fi or ethernet cable.
	  ■ Test connection prior to visit (if possible).

Privacy/ security	• Use a secure, HIPAA-compliant platform.
	• Provider location
	  ■ Conduct visits from a private space.
	  ■ Use headphones with a microphone; never use speakerphone.
	  ■ Inform the patient if others are present (e.g., students, team members).
	  ■ Check patient ID.
	• Patient location
	  ■ Confirm emergency contact information and location of patient.
	  ■ Clarify those present for visit.
	  ■ Confirm permission for their participation.
	  ■ Confirm consent.

Data from: Kelli Garber, Tina Gustin, and Carolyn Rutledge, Selection from "Put PEP into Telehealth: An Etiquette Framework for Successful Encounters," *OJIN: The Online Journal of Issues in Nursing*, vol. 28, no. 2.

In addition to adding virtual nursing and therapeutic communication content into nursing programs, nurse educators can role model the applicable essentials of netiquette of PEP in their actions with students in synchronous online classes, in online video meetings, and during virtual office hours. In addition, nurse educators can provide online practice for students using simulated experiences and incorporate telehealth communication and etiquette skills for application to the virtual setting (Taylor & Fuller, 2021).

Telehealth Empathy

Empathy is a vital component of nursing and health care in any setting, and the virtual setting is no different. The absence of face-to-face interaction, ineffective technology, and lack of a physical presence are challenges that can impact the display of empathy by the provider; healthcare providers must work to overcome the challenges in a virtual healthcare setting (Budd et al., 2022). In addition to physical displays of empathy, such as nodding, slow speech, gentle tone, and conversation pauses (see Table 8.1), the Institute for Healthcare Improvement (IHI) suggests providers use the mnemonic SAVE to ensure empathetic verbal communication:

> S for support—Let's work together to figure out what to do next. I'm here to answer all your questions. How can I help?
>
> A for acknowledge—You look like maybe you have questions. I can see that this is hard for you.
>
> V for validation—Many people feel that talking like this can feel a little awkward. Let's try to make it work.
>
> E for emotion naming—You seem worried. Help me understand how you feel right now.
>
> (Perez-Protto, 2021, para. 8)

It is important for the telehealth provider to listen beyond the words to determine what the silence conveys and to take a deeper look at what questions the patient really has. Then the provider can follow up with questions about health needs and acknowledgment of the patient's concerns using the SAVE cues from IHI.

SHOW WHAT YOU KNOW ASSIGNMENT

Imagine you are engaged in a telehealth visit with a seemingly shy, quiet patient who seems reluctant to share information. Read the article below about empathy and then answer the following questions.

1. How could you as the virtual nurse "dig deeper" to determine the patient's feelings, concerns, and health issues?
2. How would you apply the key pieces of the acronym "EMPATHY" from the article to the telehealth situation?
3. Discuss any additional online communication, empathy, and netiquette skills that you could or would use in this situation.

Article: Hofmann, P. B. (2020). Empathy's role in improving resiliency: Genuine compassion can help heal staff members and patients. *Healthcare Executive, 35*(4), 28–29.

Empathy's Role in Improving Resiliency

Genuine compassion can help heal staff members and patients.

Paul B. Hofmann, DrPH, LFACHE

Given the unprecedented impact of the coronavirus pandemic, accelerating steps needed to elevate empathetic behavior is especially important. A psychologically safe and just culture will assist staff and patients in coping more effectively when uncertainty and fear are so ubiquitous. There is no panacea, but each incremental effort will be worth the investment.

In her notable 2013 TED Talk, Harvard professor and psychiatrist Helen Riess, MD, provides several breathtaking examples of human empathy (see sidebar below). During the talk Riess says, "The good news about empathy is that when it declines, it can also be learned. Employers who want to have an engaged and productive workforce need to get tuned into the people. Patients who don't feel cared about have longer recovery rates and poor immune function."

During an extended phone conversation I had with Riess early this year, she emphasized that the qualities of empathy are teachable and, eventually, lead to an improvement in staff attitudes and behavior.

More recently, she told me, "During the COVID-19 pandemic, empathy is needed more than ever at every level of healthcare organizations. Our patients need greater empathy because of the increased threats to their safety, and our colleagues need support and permission to ask for help that may be difficult for them."

The Power of Empathy

Harvard professor and psychiatrist Helen Riess, MD, works at Massachusetts General Hospital and is the co-founder, chief scientist and chair of Empathetics Inc. Her remarkable 2013 TED Talk, "The Power of Empathy," has been viewed over 500,000 times.

During the talk, Riess mentions having received a request from one of her students who wanted to determine if, when there is empathy between people, their heart rates and other physiological tracers become concordant. The student also wanted to recruit doctor-patient pairs who were willing to have their sessions videotaped and be hooked up to monitoring devices during those sessions. Riess approved the project, participated in it and, in the TED Talk, explains how she became a more effective therapist as a result of analyzing the videos. According to Riess, the familiar statement, "I feel your pain," is actually validated by neuron studies of the brain.

This experience led her to learn everything she could about the neuroscience of empathy which, in turn, motivated her to develop empathy training grounded in the neurobiology of emotions and empathy. The training was evaluated in a randomized control trial where those doctors trained in empathy were reported by patients as being better listeners, showing more compassion and better understanding patient concerns.

Riess created the acronym E-M-P-AT-H-Y to help us remember the key pieces of how we connect to people. In the TED Talk, she describes:

- The "E" represents eye contact. Every human being, Riess says, "has a longing to be seen, understood and appreciated."
- The "M" represents facial expression muscles. Riess suggests our faces are actually a road map of human emotion that can rarely be completely hidden.
- The "P" represents posture. Riess indicates "posture is another powerful conveyor of connection." She cites a widely publicized study (*Journal of Pain and Symptom Management*, May 2005) in which researchers at MD Anderson Cancer Center in Houston found that physicians who were asked to sit down when making rounds in a patient's room were rated as being much warmer and more caring and were estimated to have spent three to five times longer with their patients than doctors who remained standing, even though both sets of physicians spent the same amount of time with patients.

- The "A" represents affect. Physicians are trained to evaluate a patient's affect as a way of assessing the person's emotional state.
- The "T" represents tone of voice. According to Riess, the nuclei for tone of voice and facial expression reside in the same area of our brain stems. "This means that when we are emotionally activated, our tone of voice and our facial expressions change without our even trying," Riess says. With practice, Riess notes, we can become more capable of hearing and seeing what these emotions are.
- The "H" represents hearing the whole person. "Far more than the words that people say, hearing the whole person means understanding the context in which other people live," Riess says.
- The "Y" represents one's response to others' feelings. "We respond to other people's feelings all the time," Riess says. "We might think that we only experience our own emotions, but we're constantly absorbing the feelings of others."

The Importance of Unhurried Conversations

The article "Careful and Kind Care Requires Unhurried Conversations," published in the Oct. 29, 2019, issue of *NEJM Catalyst*, highlights a similar theme. According to the authors, "To enable unhurried conversations, whether face-to-face, via telemedicine, asynchronous or virtual, participants need to make themselves cognitively and emotionally available."

Any program that promotes empathy and benefits patients as well as staff by increasing their resiliency in the face of pandemics, illness, trauma or occupational stress should be pursued vigorously.

It is true that the term "unhurried conversations" implies that such discussions will take more time than perhaps is desired when there are intense pressures on clinicians to increase productivity, see more patients and become more efficient. However, reality and perception are not always aligned. This familiar adage was confirmed by five noteworthy articles: the previously cited 2005 issue of the *Journal of Pain and Symptom Management*; a 2011 issue of *Patient Education and Counseling*; a 2016 issue of the *Patient Experience Journal*; a 2016 issue of the *Journal of Hospital Medicine*; and a 2017 issue of the *Journal of Nursing Care Quality*. Each article reported the results of studies that consistently demonstrated that patients perceived doctors and nurses spending more time with them than other clinicians when the staff member simply sat down.

In an article I co-authored with Jeffrey Selberg in the January/February 2006 issue of *Healthcare Executive*, we recommended several steps that should be taken to promote a culture of empathy. At least three deserve re-emphasis:

- Establish objective performance indicators, standards and goals regarding patient-centered care; monitor results; and routinely report findings to senior management, medical staff leadership and board members.
- Create opportunities for patients and family members to promote quality healthcare and improve workflow processes by serving on hospital advisory committees.
- Insist that senior executives make regular patient rounds to remind them of the value of interacting directly with patients and staff on clinical units.

Given our experience with COVID-19, we know resources and time are going to be insufficient to meet the needs of every clinician. Consequently, any program that promotes empathy and benefits patients as well as staff by increasing their resiliency in the face of pandemics, illness, trauma or occupational stress should be pursued vigorously.

Conclusion

Virtual nursing for continuous hospital care and telehealth for episodic healthcare visits may be associated with some challenges; however, both nurses and patients benefit from and are satisfied with virtual nursing and telehealth. The art of nursing in the virtual practice world requires attention to caring actions, empathy, and presence specifically because the virtual nurse-patient encounter is important to the positive health outcome of the patient. Online nurse educators should consider the inclusion of virtual nursing and telehealth nursing care into all levels of nursing curricula with a particular emphasis on caring and therapeutic communication skills. In addition, online nurse educators are positioned to role model these caring skills for transfer to the virtual nursing practice setting. In addition, the chapter provided suggestions for how to employ caring actions and therapeutic communication skills to inform the practice of nurses, APRNs, and nurse educators.

TAKE 5

List five take-away points from Chapter 8.

What did you learn?

1.
2.
3.
4.
5.

What additional information do you need to understand the concepts? See the Chapter Resources for additional material.

CHAPTER ACTIVITIES

1. Read the article "Empathy and Gratitude" under the "Show What You Know Assignment." Answer the questions associated with the article.
2. Create a telehealth caring presence and empathy plan. What question prompts are important to you for use in a telehealth encounter as the virtual healthcare provider? How would you set up your home or work office environment to accommodate telehealth visits or virtual nursing actions?
3. Continue with your long-term self-care plan and weekly journal entries.

CHAPTER RESOURCES

1. American Telemedicine Association: https://www.americantelemed.org
2. Center for Connected Health Policy (CCHP), Understanding Telehealth Policies: https://www.cchpca.org
3. HealthIT government website, Frequently Asked Questions: https://www.healthit.gov/faqs

For more information on telehealth:

4. Marquez, J. (2021). How the telehealth trend is revolutionizing medical care as we know it. *Johnson & Johnson*: https://www.jnj.com/innovation/how-telehealth-is-revolutionizing-medical-care
5. National Consortium of Telehealth Resource Centers (TRC): https://telehealthresourcecenter.org

REFERENCES

American Nurses Association. (2021). *What is nursing: The definition of nursing.* https://www.nursingworld.org/practice-policy/workforce/what-is-nursing/

Auerbach, D., Buerhaus, P., Donelan, K., & Staiger, D. (2022, August, 13). A worrisome drop in the number of young nurses. *Health Affairs.* https://www.healthaffairs.org/content/forefront/worrisome-drop-number-young-nurses

Barbosa-Angles, L., & Hamilton, H. M. (2020, September 22). A qualitative analysis of factors of human connection present during telehealth visits: Exploring and developing the concept of telepresence. *Journal of Informatics Nursing*, *5*(4), 6.

Bean, M. (2024, April, 1). The nursing workforce in 21 numbers. *Becker's Clinical Leadership.* https://www.beckershospitalreview.com/nursing/the-nursing-workforce-in-21-numbers

Board on Health Care Services, Institute of Medicine. (2012). *The evolution of telehealth: Where have we been and where are we going?* [The Role of Telehealth in an Evolving Health Care Environment: Workshop Summary]. National Academies Press.

Browne, T., McKinney, S. H., Duck, L., Baliko, B., Blake, E. W., Bethel, S. R., & Christopher, R. (2022). An academic-community interprofessional telehealth online training partnership: Impact on students and providers. *Journal of Interprofessional Care, 36*(5), 643–650. https://doi.org/10.1080/13561820.2021.1967896

Budd, G., Griffiths, D., Howick, J., Vennik, J., Bishop, F. L., Durieux, N., & Everitt, H. A. (2022). Empathy in patient-clinician interactions when using telecommunication: A rapid review of the evidence. *PEC Innovation, 1.* https://doi-org/10.1016/j.pecinn.2022.100065

Butzner, M., & Cuffee, Y. (2021) . Telehealth interventions and outcomes across rural communities in the United States: Narrative review. *Journal of Medical Internet Research, 23*(8), e29575. https://doi.org/10.2196/29575

Carroll, K. (2018). Transforming the art of nursing: Telehealth technologies. *Nursing Science Quarterly, 31*(3), 230–232. https://doi.org/10.1177/0894318418774930

Chike-Harris, K. E., Garber, K., & Derouin, A. (2021). Telehealth educational resources for graduate nurse faculty. *Nurse Educator, 46*(5), 295–299. https://doi.org/10.1097/NNE.0000000000001055

Delaney, M. (2022, September 1). Patient-centered care: The rise of the virtual nurse. *HealthTech.* https://healthtechmagazine.net/article/2022/09/rise-virtual-nurse

Gajarawala, S. N., & Pelkowski, J. N. (2021). Telehealth benefits and barriers. *Journal for Nurse Practitioners, 17,* 218–221. https://doi.org/10.1016/j.nurpra.2020.09.013

Garber, K., Gustin, T., & Rutledge, C. (2023). Put PEP into telehealth: an etiquette framework for successful encounters. *Online Journal of Issues in Nursing, 28*(2). https://doi.org/10.3912/OJIN.Vol28No02PPT16

Hashim, M. J. (2017). Patient-centered communication: Basic skills. *American Family Physician, 95*(1), 29–34.

HCA Healthcare. (2024, March 6). How virtual nursing is increasing nurse satisfaction and transforming patient care. *HCA Healthcare Today,* https://hcahealthcaretoday.com/2024/03/06/how-virtual-nursing-is-increasing-nurse-satisfaction-and-transforming-patient-care/

Health IT.Gov. (2019). *Frequently asked questions.* https://www.healthit.gov/faq/why-telehealth-important-rural-providers

Health Resources and Services Administration. (2022) *Health workforce: Nurse workforce projections, 2020–2035.* [Fact sheet]. https://bhw.hrsa.gov/sites/default/files/bureau-health-workforce/Nursing-Workforce-Projections-Factsheet.pdf

Henry, B. W., Block, D. E., Ciesla, J. R., McGowan, B. A., & Vozenilek, J. A. (2017). Clinician behaviors in telehealth care delivery: A systematic review. *Advances in Health Sciences Education, 22*(4), 869–888. https://doi.org/10.1007/s10459-016-9717-2

Herrera, A., & Foronda, C. (2022). From bedside to webside: Telehealth education for doctoral nursing students. *Journal of Doctoral Nursing Practice, 15*(3), 165–172. https://doi.org/10.1891/JDNP-2021-0049

Koehne, K. (2023). Empathy and gratitude in telehealth. *Viewpoint, 45*(4), 12–13. American Academy of Ambulatory Care Nursing.

Loughlin, B. (2023, July, 18). *Virtual nursing: The radical transformation of the way nurses work.* [Webinar]. American Nursing Informatics Association. https://library.ania.org/conferences/1/view

Love, R. & Carrington, J. (2021). Introducing telehealth skills into the Doctor of NursingPractice curriculum. *Journal of the American Association of Nursing Practitioners, 33*(11), 1030-1034. https://doi/10.1097/JXX.0000000000000505

National Council of State Boards of Nursing. (2024). The NCSBN 2024 environmental scan: Every moment matters, realizing lasting impact. *Journal of Nursing Regulation, 14*(Supplement), S1–S41.

Office of the National Coordinator for Health Information Technology. (2023). *HealthITgov: Frequently asked questions.* https://www.healthit.gov/faq/why-telehealth-important-rural-providers

Perez-Protto, S. (2021). Tips for expressing empathy via telemedicine. [Interview.]. *Insights.* Institute for Healthcare Improvement. https://www.ihi.org/insights/tips-expressing-empathy-telemedicine

Poirier, A. (2023, January, 12). Trinity Health examines in-hospital virtual care model. *Crain's Grand Rapids Business.* https://www.crainsgrandrapids.com/news/health-care/trinity-health-examines-in-hospital-virtual-care-model/

Pravecek, B., Callies, D., & Arends, R. (2024). Telehealth and teleradiology: What you need to know. *Journal of Radiology Nursing, 43*(1), 75–78. https://doi-org/10.1016/j.jradnu.2023.09.008

Rambur, B., Val Palumbo, M., & Nurkanovic, M. (2019). Prevalence of telehealth in nursing: Implications for regulation and education in the era of value-based care. *Policy, Politics, & Nursing Practice, 20*(2) 64–73. https://doi.org/10.1177/1527154419836752

Rettinger, L., & Kuhn, S. (2023). Barriers to video call-based telehealth in allied health professions and nursing: Scoping review and mapping process. *Journal of Medical Internet Research, 25*, e46715. https://doi.org/10.2196/46715

Sanford, K., Schuelke, S., Lee, M., & Mossburg, S. E. (2023, August 30). Virtual nursing: Improving patient care and meeting workforce challenges. *PSNet*. https://psnet.ahrq.gov/perspective/virtual-nursing-improving-patient-care-and-meeting-workforce-challenges

Scurlock, C. (2023, October 6). Inpatient healthcare delivery: The emergence of virtual-first strategy. *Forbes*. https://www.forbes.com/sites/forbesbusinesscouncil/2023/10/06/inpatient-healthcare-delivery-the-emergence-of-virtual-first-strategy/?sh=4019747a527a

Taylor, J., & Fuller, B. (2021). The expanding role of telehealth in nursing: considerations for nursing education. *International Journal of Nursing Education Scholarship, 18*(1). https://doi.org/10.1515/ijnes-2021-0037

Vranas, K. C., Slatore, C. G., & Kerlin, M. P. (2018). Telemedicine coverage of intensive care units: A narrative review. *Annals of the American Thoracic Society, 15*(11), 1256–1264. https://doi-org/10.1513/AnnalsATS.201804-225CME

Wicklund, E. (2023, October 4). Hospitals are looking for hard ROI in virtual nursing. *Healthleaders*. https://www.healthleadersmedia.com/technology/hospitals-are-looking-hard-roi-virtual-nursing

Wochcieckowski, M. (2023, August 7). Nurses as key players in telehealth. [Blog.]. *Daily Nurse*. https://dailynurse.com/nurses-as-key-players-in-telehealth/

Credits

Table 8.1: Kelli Garber, Tina Gustin, and Carolyn Rutledge, Selection from "Put PEP into Telehealth: An Etiquette Framework for Successful Encounters," *OJIN: The Online Journal of Issues in Nursing*, vol. 28, no. 2. Copyright © 2023 by American Nurses Association. Reprinted with permission.

Icon 8.1: Owl icon is Copyright © by Microsoft.

Icon 8.2: Copyright © by Microsoft.

Icon 8.3: Pencil icon is Copyright © by Microsoft.

Icon 8.4: Computer icon is Copyright © by Microsoft.

CHAPTER 9

Self-Care for Online Nursing Educators and Virtual Nurses

"When you take care of yourself, you're a better person for others. When you feel good about yourself, you treat others better."

—SOLANGE KNOWLES (AMERICAN SINGER-SONGWRITER, ACTRESS)

TERMS TO KNOW

complementary health practices: Nontraditional treatments such as acupuncture, aromatherapy, massage, herbal remedies, etc.

integrative health practice: A holistic approach to healthcare that uses complementary health practices in conjunction with traditional medical therapies.

occupational burnout: The result of unhandled, chronic stress in the work setting, also known as *compassion fatigue*.

resilience: The ability to recover from difficulties and having persistence.

self-care: The practice of intentional nursing actions of nurturing self to prevent consequences of stress and burnout in order to strengthen resilience.

sisu: Finnish term that represents a "deeper reserve of power within us."

stress: A state of anxiety or worry prompted by a challenging situation; the presence of stress symptoms represents how the body reacts to pressure or changes.

telework: Work that occurs from home using electronic devices to access the internet, email, and phone to implement job responsibilities; synonymous with *remote online work*.

work–life balance: Engaging in habits that promote equal portions of rest, work, family life, and leisure; also known as *lifestyle balance.*

Chapter Overview and Objectives

This chapter provides information about the use of self-care strategies for faculty, students, and nurses engaged in the virtual work of teaching, learning, and practicing remotely. Evidence about the physical and psychological stress of remote work in the online environment for both students and faculty is presented. Learners develop a long-term self-care plan that incorporates behaviors to minimize stress and maximize work in the online environment and includes actions to promote work–life balance. Methods for role modeling positive practices for well-being in the online environment are presented.

In this chapter, the learner will:

1. Identify the physical risks of prolonged online exposure.
2. Identify the psychological risks of prolonged online exposure.
3. Examine effective strategies to minimize stress while working and learning online.
4. Plan strategies to work efficiently in the online environment.
5. Develop a long-term self-care plan that assimilates healthy practices.
6. Discuss ways to role model positive practices for well-being in the virtual setting.

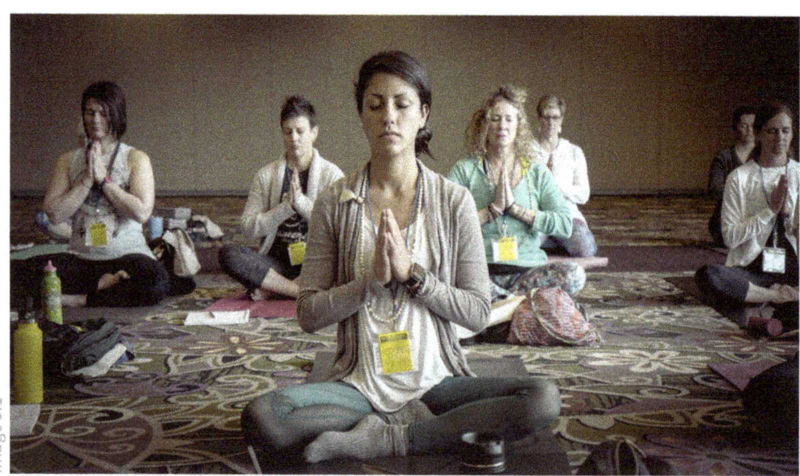

Image 9.1

Stress and Strain in the Virtual World

General Stress and Symptoms

Everyone experiences stress at some time or another. Stress is a state of anxiety or worry prompted by a challenging circumstance (World Health Organization [WHO], 2024b). The symptoms of stress can be psychological, physiological, or physical and are determined by how the body reacts to the challenging situation or change. In other words, how a person responds to stress can impact health and well-being. Short-term stress, known as situational stress, can be positive and/or motivational and urges a person to address those small challenges that occur in everyday life. Long-term stress, or chronic stress, can be detrimental to physical and mental health due to the prolonged activation of stress hormones and can cause a variety of physical and mental health problems, including anxiety, depression, gastrointestinal issues, headaches, muscle tension and pain, cardiovascular disease, myocardial infarction, hypertension, stroke, sleep problems, weight gain, and memory and concentration impairment (American Psychological Association, 2022). In addition, the use of alcohol and/or drugs to buffer stress may intensify existing health problems (National Center for Complementary and Integrative Health, 2024).

Stress in Nursing Practice

Stress in nursing practice is not new; however, the challenges associated with the COVID-19 pandemic exacerbated existing workplace problems that remain in the post-COVID-19 era. Nurses are stressed due to high patient-to-nurse ratios, low pay, lack of experienced leadership, feeling undervalued, increased incivility in the workplace, and the nursing shortage crisis (American Nurses Association [ANA], 2023). The National Council State Boards of Nursing predicts that the current nursing shortage of around 100,000 will increase by 900,000 by 2027 (NCSBN, 2023). Occupational burnout is the result of unhandled, chronic stress in any workplace setting and manifests in three dimensions: "feelings of energy depletion or exhaustion, increased mental distance from one's job or feelings of negativism or cynicism related to one's job, and reduced professional efficacy" (WHO, 2024b, para. 3). The identified stressors and feelings of burnout cause nurses to leave the profession, which further compounds the workforce shortage.

To relieve the pressures and stressors in the current nursing work environment, healthcare agencies are looking for different models of nursing care, including virtual nursing. Virtual nurses are available via computer or other electronic device to offer expertise to patients and the healthcare team and to provide appropriate documentation for nursing activities, such as patient admission, teaching, and discharge paperwork. See Chapter 8 for a complete discussion of virtual nursing. Virtual nurses may not experience the same pressures as those providing in-person nursing care, but they could be at risk for facing the physical and mental stressors associated with sedentary online remote work.

Faculty Stress

In general, university faculty face stressors due to the demands of the job, especially those in tenure-track positions who must meet the requirements for professional service, scholarship, and excellence in teaching within a specified timeframe. In addition to the demands discussed earlier, stressors for nursing faculty include instructor shortages (American Association of Colleges of Nursing [AACN], 2024), workload issues (Farber et al., 2020), revision of nursing curriculum due to changing accreditation standards, clinical supervision of students, finding time for clinical nursing practice to maintain certification (Thomas et al., 2019), and keeping current with best practice initiatives. Other important factors that cause stress and burnout specifically for nurse faculty are listed in Box 9.1. The current severe nursing shortage (NCSBN, 2023) places additional stressors on faculty to recruit and retain students for entry into the profession.

Online Faculty Stress: COVID-19 and Beyond

COVID-19

Stress factors impacting faculty during the COVID-19 pandemic were related to the fast transfer of face-to-face courses to an online format, student issues, and lack of instructor knowledge (Cothran et al., 2023). For university faculty who remained satisfied with online teaching during the pandemic, the most pertinent factors for faculty well-being were tied to a quality work environment that included reasonable workload and working conditions, technology factors, job satisfaction (Mosquera et al., 2022), and self-care to support resiliency (Riess et al., 2023). Resiliency is the ability to recover from difficulties and having persistence.

BOX 9.1 Additional Causes of Stress Leading to Nurse Faculty Burnout

- Lack of orientation to the faculty role
- Student issues (e.g., attitudes, incivility, academic dishonesty)
- Lack of university support (e.g., administrative duties, mentoring, collaboration)
- Lack of personal–professional life balance
- Faculty-to-faculty incivility
- Poor work–life balance
- Inadequate sleep, diet, and exercise
- Unrealistic professional goals

Adapted from: Thomas, C. M., Bantz, D. L., & McIntosh, C. E. (2019). Nurse faculty burnout and strategies to avoid it. *Teaching and Learning in Nursing*, *14*(2), 111–116. https://doi.org/10.1016/j.teln.2018.12.005

Nursing faculty also reported significant stress and burnout due to the COVID-19 pandemic (Leaver et al., 2022) and a decrease in well-being (Sacco & Kelly, 2021). Specifically, nurse faculty reported increases in stress and anxiety associated with switching to a virtual environment, concern about acquiring the virus, lack of support from university administration, constant changes in policies, and physical and emotional fatigue (Riess et al., 2023). Faculty also experienced anxiety and fatigue related to listening to students' COVID stories and providing support during this time (Orth & Evenson, 2023). For the post-COVID-19 future, AACN leaders recommend that nursing education entities "provide necessary resources for educators, students, and practicing nurses to optimize virtual environments to enhance education and health outcomes for all" (Leaver et al., 2022, p. 87).

Post COVID-19: Physical and Emotional Effects of Remote Work

While the anxiety and strain associated with confronting the pandemic has waned, stressors exist for those faculty who continue to teach online and for virtual nurses who work remotely. Other terms associated with remote work/online teaching are *working from home* or *telework*. Higher amounts of weekly time working from home may be associated with more stress-related symptoms and may negatively influence job satisfaction (Niebuhr et al., 2022). Prolonged sitting at a computer has implications for health; for example, decreased movement due to sedentary work may result in neck, muscle, and joint pain; weight gain; and chronic mental health problems (Atrium Health, n.d.; Hanna et al., 2023). Additionally, remote workers may suffer from sleep disorders and mental health issues (Afonso et al., 2021) and eye strain associated with viewing a computer screen for extended periods. Employees working from home lack the comradery and conversation that exist in the in-person work setting, and the stressors may be compounded due to the isolation (Urwin, 2023); supervisors can assist with decreasing the loneliness associated with working remotely (Montanez, 2024) through online meetings to check on well-being and to bring colleagues together for conversation and socialization. By having this knowledge, online nurse faculty can promote self-care for students in the virtual teaching–learning environment.

Work–Life Balance

Adequate work–life balance is associated with nurse satisfaction in the practice setting (Williams et al., 2022). Work–life balance involves engagement in activities that support equitable portions of rest, work, family time, and leisure in one's life. Maintaining work–life balance is just as important for remote workers/online faculty as for in-person employees. Remote work has some built-in flexibility; however, online faculty may be hindered by increased workload due to time spent preparing teaching materials and technological issues (Elshami et al., 2021) that can prolong the workday and interfere with family and leisure time.

Strategies to Minimize Stress and Promote Work–Life Balance

All health-related self-care activities should be managed in consultation with a primary healthcare provider. Engaging in self-care is a skill set, and evidence-based interventions can positively impact a nurse's work–life balance (Williams et al., 2022). For the purposes of this chapter, *self-care* is defined as the practice of intentional nursing actions of self nurturing to prevent consequences of stress and burnout in order to strengthen resilience. Additionally, online faculty must practice activities of self-care to remain healthy for students and others requiring attention and care (Cicco, 2020). The three main actions to minimize stress symptoms and preserve a healthy work–life balance are getting adequate rest, maintaining a nutritious diet, and engaging in healthy exercise. Other examples of self-care actions, known as complementary and integrative health (CIH) practices, are shown in Table 9.1.

Broad actions related to three main areas may involve discussions with a dietician about healthy food choices, appointments with a healthcare provider about sleep and other stress-related symptoms, and meetings with a personal trainer to develop a fitness plan. Online faculty and virtual nurses can engage with online videos from reputable organizations for more information about sleep, diet, and exercise. Self-care apps provide reminders and tracking for self-care actions; some apps provide activities like prompts for relaxation activities and breathing exercises. Examples of free wellness apps developed specifically for nurses are Nursewell, which includes actions to promote improved sleep, back health, mindfulness, well-being, clearer thinking, and better eating habits, and FifthWindow, which includes reminders and tips for self-care and fosters connections with others. Both are available at online app stores.

Sitting at a computer to perform one's responsibilities as online faculty or virtual nursing is sedentary work, which is associated with numerous health risks and injuries, as discussed earlier in the chapter. In addition to the activities to maintain a stable work–life balance, such as rest, diet, and exercise, other self-care actions can also support safety and health throughout the workday. See the *Teacher Tidbits* for some fast, time-friendly behaviors to decrease the effects of prolonged sitting and isolation while working from home.

TABLE 9.1 Complementary and Integrative Health Activities to Decrease Stress

Activities	Definition	Action	For More information
Yoga	Involves postures, poses, and breathing techniques	Combines movement with meditative techniques; associated with decreased anxiety, reduced depression, improved sleep, and many other benefits.	National Center for Complementary and Integrative Health https://www.nccih.nih.gov/health/yoga-what-you-need-to-know?nav=govd
Tia chi	Includes physical movement, imagery, and relaxed breathing	Associated with clearer thinking, decreased anxiety, reduced depression, improved sleep, and other possible benefits.	See "Tai Chi for Nurses" in Chapter Resources.
Meditation	Action that involves mental focus to promote mind–body integration.	Relaxes the mind and promotes well-being; has stress-reducing effects.	National Center for Complementary and Integrative Health https://www.nccih.nih.gov/health/meditation-and-mindfulness-what-you-need-to-know?nav=govd
Mindfulness	A form of meditation; being present in the moment	May help relieve anxiety and depression symptoms, reduce insomnia, and improve sleep quality.	National Center for Complementary and Integrative Health https://www.nccih.nih.gov/health/meditation-and-mindfulness-what-you-need-to-know?nav=govd
Relaxation techniques	Examples include deep breathing, progressive muscle relaxation, and guided imagery	Produce a sense of calmness; may help with relaxation to decrease anxiety, heart rate, and blood pressure.	National Center for Complementary and Integrative Health https://www.nccih.nih.gov/health/relaxation-techniques-what-you-need-to-know?nav=govd

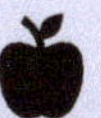

TEACHER TIDBITS FOR REMOTE WORK

Using Desk and Break Activities to Support Health

Target Area	Activities
Eyes, body, back, neck	• Place the computer screen on the desk just below eye level and set the screen an arm's length away. • Desk chair should support back and posture.
General health, diet, exercise, and rest	• Take a 1- to 2-minute break every 15 minutes and do relaxation breathing or a chair exercise. Or take 5- to 10-minute breaks every 50 minutes and take a walk, get a breath of fresh air, and drink some water. • Use a smaller water bottle; you will need to move to fill it up several times per day. • Have healthy snacks in single portions; keep snacks in the kitchen, which encourages a short walk to get them. • Schedule lunch/meal times in your daily planner; take lunch away from the desk and be mindful of the food. • Monitor daily steps; use a step counter on an app to track.
Muscle and joints	• During computer breaks, do calf stretches, finger stretches, wrist flexion, and ankle pumps.
Lower extremities	• Wear compression stockings while at the computer (15 to 20 or even 20 to 30 mm Hg) to decrease lower extremity edema (Yale Medicine, 2024).

Target Area	Activities
Overall mental health	• Keep a gratitude journal at your desk; start each workday by writing three things in the journal that you are thankful for. • Schedule a time to stop work at the end of each day. • Engage in relaxation breathing exercises several times a day.
Overall health	• Consider a sit-to-stand desk, which encourages movement and stimulates circulation.

Adapted from: Princeton University Health Services. (2024). *Ergonomics and computers*. https://uhs.princeton.edu/health-resources/ergonomics-computer-use#deskstretch; Yale Medicine. (2024).*Why sitting is so bad for us.* https://www.yalemedicine.org/news/sitting-health-risks

Nursing Education and Stress

Nursing education programs must consider the well-being of students in a high-stress health occupation such as nursing, as they are at risk for physical and mental health issues similar to nurses in practice. Registered nurse students enrolled in advanced nursing programs may present to school with existing work–life stressors. Nursing students in online programs have risks for stress symptoms similar to any person who works remotely. Additional stressors for online students in advanced nursing programs include time spent on the computer to complete course assignments coupled with balancing work, school, and family life. Nursing students in accelerated online programs are under even greater stress due to compressed course schedules.

Stress-Reducing Initiatives for Students

Educating students about work–life balance and incorporating self-care programs into nursing courses can be effective. Several nursing programs have been successful with various self-care frameworks. Green (2020) offered a 5-week self-care program to nursing students in an accelerated program; students reported a decrease in stress symptoms and an improved capability to deal with stress after completion of the program. Apsay et al. (2023) developed the Reflect, Recharge, and Revive framework (see Box 9.2); the framework starts with self-care self-awareness and concludes with sustainability ideas for personal growth and long-term goals for self-care.

BOX 9.2 Reflect, Recharge, Revive Initiative

- **Reflect:** Individualized to one's own experience with self-care.
  - Self-awareness
  - Self-reflection
- **Recharge:** Restore healthy actions for physical, mental, and spiritual well-being.
  - Self-care education and training
- **Revive:** Reflect on knowledge gained in the recharge stage; set goals and priorities for personal growth in order to be an effective professional.
  - Sustainability

Source: Apsay, K. L. G. (2023). Fostering self-care for Filipino nurse educators: A policy paper. *Philippine Journal of Nursing*, *93*(2), 66–73.

The AACN (2021) updated the Essentials for nursing education programs; the Essentials, called Domains, contain competencies for student achievement in both entry-level and advanced practice nursing education programs. Domain 10, "Personal, Professional, and Leadership Development," reflects self-care, well-being, and resiliency (see Box 9.3). Self-care and resiliency are necessary skills for nursing students to learn while in nursing school and to maintain throughout their years of practice to support their health and well-being. Students in advanced nursing programs are called upon to support a practice milieu that supports and evaluates nurse self-care and well-being in practice. Nursing programs should anticipate including opportunities in their revised curricula to meet the self-care, well-being, and resiliency competencies.

Faculty Actions to Decrease Student Stress and Increase Resiliency

Online nurse faculty can weave self-care information, assignments, and assessments throughout the curriculum. In addition, faculty can role model self-care practices in the online setting. Small actions such as checking in on students via email or through course announcements, sending reminders for self-care activities, placing relaxation and breathing exercises and calming imagery in faculty-recorded lectures and PowerPoint presentations are simple ways to encourage self-care in students. Ask students to post their favorite self-care activity in the introduction section of the course. Faculty can incorporate self-care plans into discussion board activities and place links to videos and other resources for self-care activities in the online course.

BOX 9.3 Domain 10 and Related Self-Care Competencies

Entry-Level Professional Nursing Education	Advanced-Level Nursing Education
10.1 Demonstrate a commitment to personal health and well-being.	
10.1a Demonstrate healthy, self-care behaviors that promote wellness and resiliency.	10.1c Contribute to an environment that promotes self-care, personal health, and well-being.
10.1b Manage conflict between personal and professional responsibilities.	10.1d Evaluate the workplace environment to determine level of health and well-being.

Source: American Association of Colleges of Nursing. (2021). *The Essentials: Core competencies for professional nursing education.* https://www.aacnnursing.org/Portals/0/PDFs/Publications/Essentials-2021.pdf

Resilience is the ability to recover from challenging situations. Student engagement in self-care activities fosters resilience, which may lead to better achievement of academic goals (Lin et al., 2020). Universities and faculty can support students in being resilient through interventions that assist with adapting and coping to stress. Mindfulness, praying, reading, and sleeping are associated with resilience for students in the health professions (Lin et al., 2020), which further supports the need for nursing faculty to incorporate self-care education and actions into online nursing curricula.

Sisu

One area that is gaining recognition is *sisu* (pronounced "see-soo"), a Finnish term that represents a "deeper reserve of power within us" (Mackoff, 2023), which is similar to resilience. In the book *The Leadership Laboratory*, Mackoff discusses the work of Emilia Lahti, an expert on the concept of sisu (Lahti, 2019). Sisu is described as the ability to dig deep for one's inner strength and untapped reserve to overcome a situation or challenge or to get an overwhelming job done; sisu, when used appropriately, makes one stronger (Lahti, 2019; Mackoff, 2023). Faculty can tap into the concept of resilience and digging deep into the inner self by asking students about experiences when sisu was brought forth for situations in their nursing practice. The three elements of sisu and four associated cognitive strategies are presented in Box 9.4 (Mackoff, 2023).

The ability to be resilient and/or pull from one's inner strength and demonstrate the elements of sisu in the presence of adversity may depend on one's ability to engage in self-care and healthy behaviors. Barriers that could sabotage self-care practices depend on the level of stress and burnout the nurse or nurse faculty is experiencing; major barriers are lack of motivation, being unaware of needs, misconceptions about lack of time, lack of self-worth, and not prioritizing one's needs (National Society of Health Coaches, 2023). The same barriers exist for those nurses in the

BOX 9.4 Elements with Attributes and Strategies with Actions of Sisu

Three Sisu Elements	Attributes
1. Sisu is an extraordinary perseverance.	• Complete what one has stated regardless of difficulty. • Do the impossible. • Work with integrity; no shortcuts.
2. Sisu is a latent source of reserved but not yet presented energy and power.	• Call upon one's power and energy reserve. • Act toward a vision of the end result. • Get a second wind. • Energy and resolve appear in the presence of adversity.

Three Sisu Elements	Attributes
3. Sisu is an action mindset.	• Take action despite the odds. • Demonstrate courage and hope toward challenges. • Envision success. • Change a barrier into a bridge to act. • Act creatively in the presence of hardship.

Four Cognitive Strategies	Actions
1. Discernment	• Discover meaning in reality. • Engage in reflective thinking. • Determine faith from facts.
2. Self-efficacy	• Draw upon internal strength. • Have positive belief in self to accomplish goals/outcomes. • Lead with knowledge of growth.
3. Deliberate thought	• Be mindful of intentions. • Engage in positive self-talk. • Envision outcomes.
4. Bricolage (solving problems with the resources available)	• Draw upon and create solutions with available resources. • Improvise.

Adapted from: Mackoff, B. (2023). *Leadership laboratory for nurse leaders*. Cognella.

virtual world. Nursing education and practice leaders can prioritize self-care initiatives for nurse faculty and virtual nurses by identifying and diminishing stressors in the work environment and providing time and support for healthy activities. A check-in during the beginning of a virtual meeting can set the tone for a caring supportive environment. Incorporating self-care goals into the annual performance review highlights the importance of healthy actions for everyday well-being. All nurses are encouraged to complete a self-care plan that incorporates short- and long-term goals for maintaining health and work–life balance. Review the sample self-care plan in the "Show What You Know Assignment."

SHOW WHAT YOU KNOW ASSIGNMENT

Directions: Develop a self-care plan that includes activities to support health and well-being while working online as well as actions to support work–life balance. Use chapter and resource information to complete the plan. There are examples listed under "rest/sleep" to help you get started.

a. Include daily goals for exercise, adequate diet, and sleep.
b. Include a plan to engage in positive health practices.
c. Include self-care actions for working remotely/online.
d. Incorporate activities from your self-care journal.
e. Think about the principles of sisu and your ability to get work and the self-care plan accomplished.

Remember that a little self-care is better than none at all.

(Continued)

Long-Term Goal	Rest/Sleep		Healthy Diet		Exercise		Mental Health Actions	
Goal [Example]	Maintain adequate sleep and rest		Implement a healthy plan for meals and snacks		Implement a plan for movement/ exercise		Maintain a plan for positive mental health	
Activities to Meet Goals	**Activity**	**How Often**	**Activity**	**How Often**	**Activity**	**How Often**	**Activity**	**How Often**
Activity (examples provided for rest/sleep)	Sleep 7–8 hours/day Take work breaks—see short-term goals Write breaks in planner Determine a time that work ends each day	Daily Take breaks hourly						

Short-Term Hourly Goals	Overall Health, Exercise, and Rest		Good Health for Muscles, Joints, Lower Extremities		Good Health for the Neck, Back, and Eyes		Positive Mental Health	
Self-Care Actions While Working Online	Action	How Often	Action	How Often	Action	How Often	Action	How Often
	1- to 2-minute breaks with relaxation breathing and chair exercises; *or*	Every 15 minutes						
	5- to 10-minute break; include a walk, fresh air, drink of water	Every 50 minutes						
	Monitor daily steps; use a step counter on an app to track							

Conclusion

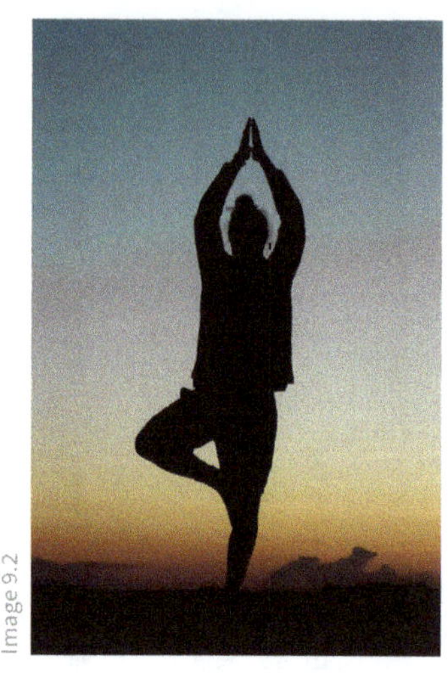
Image 9.2

Nurses in any setting have an ethical obligation to themselves to engage in self-care in order to be at their best to serve others (Linton & Koonmen, 2020) whether it be virtual or in person, in practice or in education. Alexander and Kelch (2021) who write for the newsletter *Inside Higher Ed* state, "our time is always a gift. Daily, those of us who work in higher education should purposefully attend to our important needs, even if only for a short time each day" (para. 10). Nurses who are remote workers need to schedule time each day to take breaks, refresh, and refuel, which will strengthen the resilience that is needed during challenging events. A regular routine to promote rest, a healthy diet, and adequate exercise decreases the risk of long-term physical and mental health issues.

IF YOU NEED HELP FOR MENTAL HEALTH ISSUES

If you are struggling to cope or dealing with prolonged symptoms of stress, consider meeting with a professional. If you are in immediate distress or are thinking about hurting yourself, call, text, or chat 988. This three-digit number will route you to the 988 Suicide & Crisis Lifeline, which is now active across the United States. The Lifeline provides 24-hour, confidential support to anyone in suicidal crisis or emotional distress (see https://988lifeline.org).

If you or someone you know has a mental illness, is struggling emotionally, or has concerns about their mental health, there are ways to get help. Read more at https://www.nimh.nih.gov/health/find-help/.

TAKE 5

List five take-away points from Chapter 9.

What did you learn?

1.
2.
3.
4.
5.

What additional information do you need to understand the concepts? See the Chapter Resources for additional material.

CHAPTER ACTIVITIES

1. Complete the "Show What You Know Activity Assignment" long-term plan for self-care.
2. Consider the question: What effect has taking courses online or teaching online had on your physical and emotional health? Describe the effects.
3. Describe a practice or educational challenge and explain how you demonstrated sisu in the situation.
4. **Sharing on Caring:** Keep journaling your self-care activities, note feelings, identify barriers to engaging in self-care, and add solutions for overcoming the barriers. See the form. Review your entries in the self-care journal. Celebrate your successes.

Self-Care Activity 1:									
Date									
Feelings									
Barriers									
Other Notes									

Self-Care Activity 2:									
Date									
Feelings									
Barriers									
Other Notes									

CHAPTER RESOURCES

1. American Nurses Association code of ethics and self-care—article resource: Linton, M., & Koonmen, J. (2020). Self-care as an ethical obligation for nurses. *Nursing Ethics*, 969733020940371. https://doi.org/10.1177/0969733020940371
2. American Association Colleges of Nursing tool kit for nurses for self-care: https://www.aacnnursing.org/5b-tool-kit/themes/self-care
3. American Psychological Association self-care series for psychologists; helpful for other healthcare providers: https://www.apa.org/career-development/self-care-series
4. National Center for Complementary and Integrative Health resources for mind and body health: https://content.govdelivery.com/accounts/USNIHNCCIH/bulletins/381d74a
5. American Holistic Nurses Association self-care and resilience tool kits: https://www.ahna.org/American-Holistic-Nurses-Association/Resources/Self-Care-and-Resilience
6. Miller, S. M., Hui-Lio, C., & Taylor-Piliae, R. E. (2020). Health benefits of tai chi exercise: A guide for nurses. *Nursing Clinics of North America*, *55*(4), 581–600. https://doi:10.1016/j.cnur.2020.07.002

REFERENCES

Afonso, P., Fonseca, M., & Teodoro, T. (2022). Evaluation of anxiety, depression and sleep quality in full-time teleworkers. *Journal of Public Health (Oxford, England), 44*(4), 797–804. https://doi.org/10.1093/pubmed/fdab164

Alexander, J., & Kelch, B. (2021, July 8). Self-care strategies for faculty. *Inside Higher Ed.* https://www.insidehighered.com/advice/2021/07/09/academics-should-make-time-self-care-even-if-just-few-minutes-each-day-opinion

American Association of Colleges of Nursing. (2021). *The Essentials: Core competencies for professional nursing education.* https://www.aacnnursing.org/Portals/0/PDFs/Publications/Essentials-2021.pdf

American Association Colleges of Nursing. (2022). *Nursing faculty shortage.* [Fact sheet]. https://www.aacnnursing.org/Portals/42/News/Factsheets/Faculty-Shortage-Factsheet.pdf

American Association of Colleges of Nursing. (2024). *Nursing faculty shortage.* [Fact sheet]. https://www.aacnnursing.org/news-data/fact-sheets/nursing-faculty-shortage

American Nurses Association. (2023). *Why nurses quit and leave the profession.* ANA Nurses Resources Hub. https://www.nursingworld.org/content-hub/resources/nursing-leadership/why-nurses-quit/

American Psychological Association. (2022, October 31). *How stress affects your health.* https://www.apa.org/topics/stress/health

Atrium Health. (n.d.). Working remotely can be a "pain in the neck" as well as the back and other joints. https://www.wakehealth.edu/coronavirus/stress-and-coping/working-remotely-can-be-a-pain-in-the-neck

Apsay, K. L. G. (2023). Fostering self-care for Filipino nurse educators: A policy paper. *Philippine Journal of Nursing, 93*(2), 66–73.

Cicco, G. (2020). Online instruction during a pandemic: Faculty collaboration and self-care. *I-Manager's Journal of Educational Technology, 17*(3), 1–5.

Cothran, S. L., Hegler, C. M., Martinez-Dawson, R., Dawson, P. L., & Northcutt, J. K. (2023). Faculty stress factors at a public university during the COVID-19 pandemic. *Journal of Higher Education Theory & Practice, 23*(11), 1–14. https://doi-org/10.33423/jhetp.v23i11.6214

Elshami, W., Taha, M. H., Abuzaid, M., Saravanan, C., Al Kawas, S., & Abdalla, M. E. (2021). Satisfaction with online learning in the new normal: Perspective of students and faculty at medical and health sciences colleges. *Medical Education Online, 26*(1). https://doi.org/10.1080/10872981.2021.1920090

Farber, J. E., Payton, C., & Dorney, P. (2020). Life balance and professional quality of life among baccalaureate nurse faculty. *Journal of Professional Nursing, 36*(6), 587–594. https://doi-idm.oclc.org/10.1016/j.profnurs.2020.08.010

Green, C. (2020). Teaching accelerated nursing students' self-care: A pilot project. *Nursing Open, 7,* 225–234. https://doi.org/10.1002/nop2.384

Hanna, F., You, E., & Elor-Sherif, M. (2023). Editorial: The impact of sedentary behavior and virtual lifestyle on physical and mental wellbeing: Social distancing from healthy living. *Frontiers in Public Health, 11,* 1265814. https://doi.org/10.3389/fpubh.2023.1265814

Lahti, E. (2019). Embodied fortitude: An introduction to the Finnish construct of sisu. *International Journal of Wellbeing, 9*(1), 61–82. https://doi.org/10.5502/ijw.v9i1.672

Leaver, C., Stanley, J., & Veenema T. G. (2022). Impact of the COVID-19 pandemic on the future of nursing education. *Academic Medicine, 97*(3S), S82–S89.

Lin, L. C., Chan, M., Hendrickson, S., & Zuñiga, J. A. (2020). Resiliency and self-care behaviors in health professional schools. *Journal of Holistic Nursing, 38*(4), 373–381. https://doi.org/10.1177/0898010120933487

Linton, M., & Koonmen, J. (2020). Self-care as an ethical obligation for nurses. *Nursing Ethics, 27*(8), 1694–1702. https://doi.org/10.1177/0969733020940371

Mackoff, B. (2023). *Leadership laboratory for nurse leaders.* Cognella.

Montanez, R. (2024, March 22). Remote work: Fighting loneliness on remote teams. *Harvard Business Review.* https://hbr.org/2024/03/fighting-loneliness-on-remote-teams

Mosquera, P., Albuquerque, P., & Picoto, W. N. (2022). Is online teaching challenging faculty well-being? *Administrative Sciences, 12*, 147. https://doi.org/10.3390/admsci12040147

National Center for Complementary and Integrative Health. (2024). *Press reset on stress.* [Info graph]. https://www.nccih.nih.gov/health/stress

National Council State Boards of Nursing. (2023). NCSBN research projects significant nursing workforce shortages and crisis. [News release]. https://www.ncsbn.org/news/ncsbn-research-projects-significant-nursing-workforce-shortages-and-crisis

National Society of Health Coaches. (2023, June, 12). *Self-care for practitioners: Self-care for nurses—everything you should know in 2023.* https://www.nshcoa.com/self-care-for-nurses/

Niebuhr, F., Borle, P., Börner-Zobel, F., & Voelter-Mahlknecht, S. (2022). Healthy and happy working from home? Effects of working from home on employee health and job satisfaction. *International Journal of Environmental Research and Public Health, 19*(3), 1122. https://doi.org/10.3390/ijerph19031122

Orth, S. J., & Evanson, T. A. (2024). The nurse faculty role: A lived experience of mentoring nurses while coping with anxiety during the COVID-19 pandemic. *Journal of Psychiatric & Mental Health Nursing (John Wiley & Sons, Inc.), 31*(1), 111–116. https://doi.org/10.1111/jpm.12962

Riess, D., Mersiovsky, A., & Gruhn, C, (2023). Nurse educators' perceptions and self-efficacy in response to COVID-19: A scoping review. *Nurse Educator, 48*(2), E47–E52. https://doi.org/10.1097/NNE.0000000000001342

Sacco, T. L., & Kelly, M. M. (2021). Nursing faculty experiences during the COVID-19 pandemic response. *Nursing Education Perspectives, 42*(5), 285. https://doi.org/10.1097/01.NEP.0000000000000843

Thomas, C. M., Bantz, D. L., & McIntosh, C. E. (2019). Nurse faculty burnout and strategies to avoid it. *Teaching and Learning in Nursing, 14*(2), 111–116. https://doi-org/10.1016/j.teln.2018.12.005

Urwin, W. (2023, June 28). *Working from home and depression.* Builtin. https://builtin.com/articles/working-from-home-depression

Williams, S., Furh, S., Barinas, J., & Graves, R. (2022). Self-care in nurses. *Journal of Radiologic Nursing, 41*(1), 22–27. https://doi.org/10.1016/j.jradnu.2021.11.001

World Health Organization. (2024a). *Burn-out an "occupational phenomenon.": International Classification of Diseases.* https://www.who.int/news/item/28-05-2019-burn-out-an-occupational-phenomenon-international-classification-of-diseases

World Health Organization. (2024b). *What is stress? How does it affect us?* https://www.who.int/news-room/questions-and-answers/item/stress/

Credits

IMG 9.1: Copyright © 2018 Unsplash/Erik Brolin.

Icon 9.1: Apple icon is Copyright © by Microsoft.

Icon 9.2: Owl icon is Copyright © by Microsoft.

IMG 9.2: Copyright © 2018 Unsplash/Yannic Läderach.

Icon 9.3: Copyright © by Microsoft.

Icon 9.4: Pencil icon is Copyright © by Microsoft.

Icon 9.5: Computer icon is Copyright © by Microsoft.

CHAPTER 10

Caring and Technology

The Future of Online Nursing Education and Practice

"Caring is central to the art of nursing regardless of the setting, circumstance, or century."

—L. ZAJAC

TERMS TO KNOW

artificial intelligence (AI): A technology that enables computers and machines to simulate human intelligence and problem-solving capabilities.

augmented reality (AR): Uses technology to superimpose digital content in the real-world environment and then changes the experience of the environment by providing additional information; these experiences make AR useful for education and training.

extended reality (XR): A technology that merges real and virtual environments and human–machine interactions by computer technology; combines augmented reality (AR), mixed reality (MR), and virtual reality (VR).

mixed reality: A hybrid technology of VR and AR where the user can see virtual objects in the real world and have an experience in which both the physical and virtual exist; the experience is such that the user finds it difficult to tell the difference between the virtual and the physical.

virtual reality (VR): Computer-generated reproduction of a three-dimensional image or environment that the person or user interacts with and feels immersed in the surroundings. The person uses an electronic helmet or headset with a screen and/or gloves fitted with sensors for a fully immersive experience even though the environment is artificially created.

Chapter Overview and Objectives

This chapter provides the learner with current and predicted changes for online education and virtual nursing. Advances in augmented and virtual reality, gaming, and artificial intelligence have the potential to change online nursing education as well as influence virtual nursing in the clinical realm. In the future, with the use of artificial intelligence, machines may be able to detect "feelings" and a learner's sense of awareness. This chapter explores how futuristic technologies might be used to design and deliver online nursing education, impact workforce training modalities, and influence virtual nursing practice. Ideas from thought leaders about blending nursing and technology are discussed. Students will propose ideas for online teaching in the future and for creating human nursing caring moments in this "yet to come" super-technical virtual teaching-learning and practice environment.

In this chapter, the learner will:

1. Define terms related to virtual technologies.
2. Explore how future technologies may be used to design and deliver online nursing education.
3. Discuss the influence of technological advances in the practice setting on nursing education.
4. Discuss the possible future implications of artificial intelligence in online education.
5. Explore if and how caring moments in the online environment can be preserved in the presence of futuristic technologies.

Technology Advancements: The Virtual Future for Online Education and Health Care

Technological development and expansion continue to influence online education and simultaneously impact health care and healthcare delivery. Virtual technology is revolutionizing learning for students in grade school through higher education. Faculty will need to stay current with the development of virtual technologies such as virtual reality, augmented reality, mixed reality, extended reality, and artificial intelligence to be prepared for emerging innovations. These technological advancements influence the way faculty teach nursing content in undergraduate and graduate education, particularly in the online setting now and in the future.

Virtual Reality and Education

Virtual reality (VR) is a computer-generated simulation of a three-dimensional image or environment that the person or user interacts with in such a way that they are immersed in their surroundings. The person uses an electronic helmet or headset with a screen and/or gloves or handles fitted with sensors for a fully immersive experience even though the environment is artificially constructed.

The technology creates a sense of presence in the artificial environment and provides opportunities for students to see objects and people in a virtual world; therefore, it has uses for science, health care, language, and more (Evanick, 2023). The simulated reality can be used to reproduce realistic situations that otherwise could not be created in the classroom (Evanick, 2023).

Augmented Reality and Education

Augmented reality (AR) is different from VR because with AR the real world becomes the context where virtual objects, pictures, or other items are placed. Everything the person sees, including the virtual items, are viewed in the real environment. In other words, AR uses technology to superimpose digital content in the real world, therefore changing the environment by providing additional information. These features make AR useful for education and training.

AR and VR in Education

Faculty can use both VR and AR to transform online learning by developing experiences that are engaging and interactive. Students can immerse in simulated experiences; they can "explore realistic simulations, visit historical sites virtually, conduct complex experiments, and engage in hands-on activities that were previously impossible in traditional classroom settings" (Emmy, 2023, para. 3). For example, faculty can use AR to create a lifelike patient scenario for students learning nursing care. Students use a smartphone, glasses, or a headset that provides auditory, visual, and other sensory information about the scenario. There is an increased chance for reflective learning and improved retention with the use of AR and VR in education (Spilka, 2023).

Mixed Reality

Mixed reality is a hybrid technology of VR and AR; the user can see virtual objects in the real world and have an experience where both the physical and virtual exist. The experience is such that the user finds it difficult to tell the difference. In addition, extended reality uses mixed reality to further blend the physical and virtual worlds so that users/learners can interact with virtual objects present in the real or physical environment (Emmy, 2023).

Use of VR and AR for Online Course Design: Benefits and Challenges

The use of VR and AR in the virtual setting has the potential to revolutionize the online teaching–learning environment. As of this writing, their use varies depending on phases of development and availability of equipment. There are significant benefits and some challenges when considering current and future uses of VR and AR in the online teaching-learning environment, as noted in Box 10.1.

Applications of VR and AR for Online Nursing Education

VR and AR technologies could have extensive applications for nursing as they continue to evolve. Ideas for incorporating AR and VR into the online nursing curriculum for undergraduate students include using it to

(1) understand complex scientific concepts; (2) prioritize next steps in a patient care scenario; (3) practice therapeutic communication; (4) engage virtually with patients using equipment, such as IV pumps, ventilators, insulin pumps, oxygen, etc.; (5) interact in complex patient situations; and (6) provide care for groups of patients. Online graduate students in advanced nursing programs can interact with the virtual technology for (1) primary care practice scenarios, (2) leadership challenge scenarios such as conflict resolution and lateral violence situations, (3) interaction in virtual organization board meetings, (4) leadership in epidemiologic and population health disaster and crisis situations, and (5) management of acute care scenarios.

BOX 10.1 Benefits and Challenges of VR and AR to Online Course Design and Development

Benefits

- Provides students with immersive and interactive learning experience.
  - Real-life simulations for practice.
  - Allows for mistakes in a regulated virtual setting. Examples:
    - Medical students: Practice surgery.
    - APRN students: Practice suturing.
    - Engineers: Work with machinery harmlessly for them and environment.
    - Nursing students: Practice patient care scenarios; work with healthcare equipment.
- Provides students with personalized instruction.
  - Track student progress and provide feedback.
  - Adjust the level of content difficulty.
- Provides access to experiences not possible in traditional classrooms.
  - Can virtually take students to places around the globe.
  - Consider use for service learning–type experiences in nursing.
  - Can bring objects to life.
- Supports faculty use to create interesting, interactive online presentations.

- Improves social interaction in online courses.
    - Together students can:
        - Share thoughts and concepts.
        - Problem solve.
        - Work on projects in the virtual setting.
- Facilitates gaming as teaching–learning strategy.
    - Future integration into LMS to integrate leaderboards, badges, and rewards.
    - Support beneficial competition and achievement.
    - Promote engagement and collaboration, sense of accomplishment.

Challenges

- Cost of technology: Startup, development, and maintenance.
- Lack of adequate technical support and LMS infrastructure.
- Need for large-scale accessibility of the technology for online students.
    - VR headsets, helmets, screens, etc.
- Lack of knowledge by faculty and IT.
- Accessibility challenges for students with special needs.
    - Use of the technology relies on sensory cues.
    - Provide options, not barriers to learning.
- Maintain digital well-being.
    - Data security.
    - Preserve privacy.
    - Endure ethical practices.
    - Challenges with supporting accessible, equitable, and inclusive learning environments.

Adapted from: Emmy, M., (2023). *The future of e-learning: trends and predictions for 2023 and beyond*. eLearning Industry. https://elearningindustry.com/future-of-elearning-trends-and-predictions-for-2023-and-beyond; Evanick, J. (2023, June 27). *Immersive learning: How virtual and augmented reality are transforming higher education*. eLearning Industry. https://elearningindustry.com/immersive-learning-how-virtual-and-augmented-reality-transforming-higher-education

Both graduates and undergraduates can engage in virtual service learning, language learning for healthcare providers, and cultural immersion experiences through the use of VR and AR when these opportunities are not available in person. Best practices for faculty for using technology for immersive learning experiences in the online environment are listed in Box 10.2.

BOX 10.2 Best Practices for Immersive Learning

- Identify the technological needs and resources to implement the training.
  - Ensure the technology needed (i.e., hardware and software) is available.
  - Have the ability to troubleshoot if needed.
- Prepare the learners for the training.
  - Introduce and demonstrate the technology to the students.
- Make sure the learning experience stays active, not passive.
  - Keep the activity engaging and interactionable.
- Identify activity objectives and map them to learning objectives.
  - Create the activity with the outcomes/goals in mind.
- Lean into gamification.
  - Consider healthy competition as part of the immersion.
- Build a curriculum, script, and production plan.
  - Consider the actors, props, and items needed for video making for the scenario/immersion.
- Prioritize accessibility and alternative approaches for learners with special needs or other delivery constraints.
  - Consider connectivity issues and accessibility for all; consider a scaled-down version of the activity so all students can be included.
- Create activities to evaluate comprehension and skill progress.
  - Need evaluation methods to determine achievement of outcomes.
- Evaluate the effectiveness of the course relative to learning objectives.
  - Evaluate the whole immersion activity at the end of the experience.

Henry, J. (2022, December 23). Immersive learning design today: Best practices. *eLearning Industry.* https://elearningindustry.com/immersive-learning-design-today-best-practices

Artificial Intelligence (AI)

Artificial intelligence (AI) is a technology that enables computers and machines to simulate human intelligence and problem-solving capabilities. There are four types of AI (IBM, n.d.). Type 1 relative machine and Type 2 limited memory AI were discussed in Chapter 5. Type 3, the theory of mind machine, will understand thoughts and emotions and, in turn, be able to understand others' intentions and predict behavior (Coursera, 2024). This advancement will allow AI to simulate humanlike relationships; this type of AI is currently under development (IBM, 2023). Type 4 is self-aware AI, and as theorized, would have the capability to understand itself in terms of thoughts, feelings, and emotions; this type of AI has not yet been developed (IBM, 2023) as of this writing.

Predictions for the future of AI are that sophisticated AI algorithms will tailor to educational needs through the individual assessment of the student's preferences, strengths, and weaknesses to customize the course content and assessments. This individualized approach to course blueprint and real-time redesign could improve student learning and outcomes and increase retention rates (Emmy, 2023). For example, the course could or would adjust in real time as the learner is interacting with course material and assignments; furthermore, AI-powered tutors could serve as mentors, provide support, document student development, and identify strengths and learning weakness (Emmy, 2023; Mda Training, 2023). These AI-generated systems would provide individualized services to students to ensure an educational experience that is efficient and effective. This use of AI could improve students' outcomes in the online environment and increase graduation rates in nursing programs and success rates on licensing and certification exams.

Advanced Technologies for Nursing Education and Practice

Innovations in Nursing Education

Professional nursing organizations provide funds for nurses and nurse educators to develop and apply the advance technologies in nursing situations. The Ohio State University (OSU) College of Nursing in collaboration with the OSU's College of Engineering received a grant as part of the American Nurses Foundation (ANF, 2024a) "Reimagine Nursing Initiative." The colleges work together to incorporate student competencies throughout the nursing curriculum using extended reality technology based on each student's learning needs. The AI tool focuses on nurse decision-making during crucial situations, where nurses make life-or-death decisions; the tool presents progressively complex nursing situations to students in this virtual environment. This nursing education initiative has implications for faculty, students, and future patients. For more information, refer to the Chapter Resources.

Innovations for Nursing Practice and Health Care

Advances in AR, VR, and AI have the potential to improve the workforce shortage, decrease costs, provide better access to health care, and prevent provider burnout. Chapter 8 presented several of these topics related to virtual nursing and health care.

Additional considerations for advanced technology are the "digital front door" of health care (Healthcare Dive, 2024); younger patients, born into the digital technology world, may desire a virtual entry into health care with the use of an app or online platform to engage with a virtual assistant; an AI chatbot could direct the patient to an appropriate telehealth healthcare specialist or to the right care modality faster (Healthcare Dive, 2024).

Future iterations of virtual technologies and AI will have applications in other areas of health care similar to nursing education. Healthcare organizations could use virtual patient scenarios to assess nurse competencies, provide professional development, and assist healthcare providers in practicing old and new skills and procedures safely in a controlled environment. Today, there is interest in how AI will intersect with nurses in nursing practice. In a qualitative descriptive design, Rony et al. (2024) elicited the viewpoints of nurses working in education and in practice about the future integration of AI in nursing care. Ten themes emerged from the exploratory interviews: (1) perceptions of AI readiness, (2) benefits and concerns, (3) enhanced patient outcomes, (4) collaboration and workflow, (5) human-tech balance, (6) training and skill development, (7) ethical and legal considerations, (8) AI implementation barriers,

(9) patient-nurse relationships, and (10) future vision and adaptation. The conclusions from these findings indicate that healthcare organizations will need to provide education for nurses to incorporate new skills required for AI application to nursing care (Rony et al., 2024). Healthcare technology advances will have implications for nursing education in both in-person and online teaching-learning settings.

Another ANF (2024b) grant to fund the "Reimagine Nursing Initiative" focuses on nursing practice. ChristianaCare is using the grant funds for a pilot program to use Moxi cobots (a "copartner robot") built by Diligent Robotics (2023) that use AI to free up 30 percent of nurses' time spent gathering supplies, equipment, and medications; sending specimens; and performing other tasks. Moxi is integrated with the electronic health record (EHR) and can anticipate what the nurses need; the pilot program has placed cobots on 11 nursing units with 400 nurses and, if successful, the healthcare organization plans to increase usage in the future (ANF, 2024b). As of the end of 2023, there were 100 Moxi cobots in 30 hospital systems in the United States (Diligent Robotics, 2023). For more information about the Moxi cobot, see the video links in the Chapter Resources.

Implications for Online Nursing Education

Nursing education programs will need to stay vigilant with how and when technology gets integrated into healthcare organizations so nursing students can be prepared. Some technology has not gained momentum. For example, Google Glass was created using AR to display information on command in the person's visual field; the innovation was promoted to healthcare providers as a way to quickly access patient data. The glasses were introduced to the public in 2013; discontinued in 2015 due to privacy issues, cost, and design; and then retooled for business as Enterprise Glass (Korn, 2023). In 2023, Google announced the discontinuation of the Enterprise Glass effective March 15 (Google, 2023) Whether healthcare organizations incorporate AR, VR, and AI or not, online faculty in nursing education will need stay current with what technology is infused into the practice setting as the situation is rapidly changing. Leaders in nursing education and practice will need to consider how technology will change nursing workflows and functions in the healthcare setting in the future (Frith, 2021). These future advancements and changes will need to be incorporated into nursing curricula.

Human Caring in a Future Nursing World of Technology

Technology using VR, AR, and AI appears to be here to stay. The indications for the technology may waiver, like the end of Google Glass, but digital elements of the virtual world, including robotics and machine learning, have a significant market in healthcare. In 2017, 86 percent of healthcare organizations reported use of some form of AI (Siwicki, 2017). Furthermore, the global AR and VR market in the healthcare industry was estimated at $1.57 billion in 2022 and is expected to grow by 24 percent annually (Towards Healthcare, 2022). Healthcare organizations must continuously work to prepare their workforce as the technology continues to develop and expand. Read the interview in Box 10.3 with Bre Loughlin, MSN, RN, founder and CEO of the company Nurse Disrupted, a virtual nursing technology company, as she describes how caring interfaces with virtual nurses in the technology world and how her company brings nurses to the table for decisions about technology design.

While the interview in Box 10.3 discusses how caring is inherent in the virtual platform technology company, questions emerge as the nursing profession considers how nurses can coexist with AI and AR technology in a way that safeguards the parts of nursing care that are uniquely human, such as caring and compassion. Nurses have not yet been completely replaced by robots and advanced technology, but discussions ensue about what, how, and if nurses will practice in the future (Arcega et al., 2020; Frith, 2021; Stokes & Palmer, 2020). Specifically, the questions for nurses and online nurse educators are about how to preserve the human virtues of caring and compassion and human interaction that comprise the art of nursing in tandem with the technology. The Registered Nurses' Association of Ontario (RNAO, 2020) believes that AI technology and nursing can coexist, but acknowledges that there is limited research on the topic; for example, there is little information about the effect of AI on compassion/caring and family and patient-centered care. The limited available evidence suggests that the use of AI-driven robots can be beneficial to patients in some settings and does allow nurses to have more time with the patient to care for their needs (RNAO, 2020). Johnson and Carrington (2023) posit that technology could be adopted as a fifth domain into the nursing paradigm of nursing, health, person, and environment, and, through research, scholarship, and evidence-based practice, proactively determine where and how technology enhances holistic, patient-centered care. The time is now for nurses to take a more active position, ensuring holistic and patient-centered care through involvement in design of and policy creation about the use of technology to meet patients' health needs (Rubeis, 2021).

BOX 10.3 Interview with CEO Bre Loughlin

Question: How are caring and compassion incorporated within the technology and technology platforms that you use?

Bre: Caring and compassion are used and expected in all aspects of engagement within the team/company members and with our clients. Everyone at Nurse Disrupted takes part in the caring training, including the tech team. I believe that you have to give compassion to get compassion. Caring must be infused into all areas/aspects of nursing practice, including virtual nursing, to be transformative. A way to demonstrate caring is that the company includes the nurse in the development of technology. Nurse[s] are the best source for how to work around technology that does not work for them, so we make them part of the process to ensure that the technology works for the nurses who use the virtual platforms.

Question: How is caring and compassion demonstrated using the technology in the virtual setting?

Bre: One should come to the virtual setting as you would to the in-person setting: dress professionally, provide a quiet confidential environment, bring your nursing skill set and caring that you practice in the in-person setting to the virtual setting.

Question: What do you think are challenges associated with virtual nursing?

Bre: The challenges with virtual nursing are the variations in practice; consistency in nursing practice is needed regardless of the technology. The nurse needs to practice consistently whether at the bedside or virtually. I believe that all virtual nurses need experience in nursing at the bedside first.

Question: What suggestions do you have relative to virtual nursing for the nursing education curriculum?

Bre: Introduce undergraduate students to virtual nursing and then they can learn to work on a team with a virtual nurse. But first, students need some practice experience in person at the bedside. Also, virtual nurses are present [available] for more people than in-person nurses; new grads and students can rely on the experience and expertise of virtual nurses. As the new grad acquires experience, then they can add virtual nursing to their practice.

What this means for nursing education is that the curricula and nurse educators are challenged to prepare students to be digitally ready for practice along with valuing the soft skills that support patient-centered, holistic care. The nurse-patient human interaction is the mechanism for nurses to identify unique patient needs for individualized care to ensure best patient outcomes. Online nurse faculty have the additional challenge of emphasizing these soft skills in a virtual teaching-learning environment where the teaching/teachers may be replaced or at least changed by the use of technology. Online faculty should use every opportunity with online video, text, email, phone, and course feedback as a teachable moment about caring, compassion, and human connection in the presence of increasing technology. Online nursing students have opportunities to be in the best situations for learning with the use of technology, learning how technology will change nursing care delivery and still hold onto what makes us uniquely human.

Conclusion

Whether the technology is AR, VR, or AI in the online environment or in the nursing practice environment, the nurse educator can preserve, role model, and represent the human elements of caring, compassion, and presence. Online educators can stay abreast of technology and still care for students using principles of human interactions and best practices in online teaching. To keep this all in perspective, educator and journalist Nathan Pitts reminds us about the value of ourselves as people. He says,

> Take a look at your classroom and see if you can identify where *you* are in it. As Roose [author and journalist, https://www.

kevinroose.com/bio] says, "The most valuable skills and abilities [are] the ones that [can] *distinguish* workers from machines." We can never be faster or more comprehensive than AI. But it is our responsibility to be unabashedly, unreservedly, conspicuously human. (Pitts, 2023, para. 22, 23)

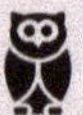

SHOW WHAT YOU KNOW ASSIGNMENT

1. Review your course map. What online assignments or course activities could benefit from the use of technology such as AI, AR, and AV?
2. What ideas do you have to infuse caring actions in a high-tech virtual world of nursing education and practice?
3. Given the current use of robots and technology in health care and how rapidly the technology is advancing, do you believe that technology such as robots could replace the work of nurse educators? Nurses at the bedside? In advanced practice nursing? Why or why not? Support your statements with evidence from the literature.

TAKE 5

List five take-away points from Chapter 10.

What did you learn?

1.
2.
3.
4.
5.

What additional information do you need to understand the concepts? See the Chapter Resources for additional material.

CHAPTER ACTIVITIES

1. Complete the "Show What You Know Assignment."
2. As an online educator, how could you ensure a place at the decision table to provide input into the design to advance the technology (AI, AR, VR, XR) for online nursing education?
3. Complete the weekly self-care journal. How did you do with your activity? What are your plans to continue with the self-care activity in the future?
4. Evaluate your progress with the long-term plan to care for yourself as a remote worker. What barriers prevent you from following the long-term plan? What are your plans to meet your goals long term?

CHAPTER RESOURCES

1. More about robotics:
   American Nurses Association. (2023). *Driving nursing outcomes through robotics*. YouTube. https://www.youtube.com/watch?v=-lcqGcZOFGA&t=41s

   Diligent Robotics. (2018). *'Moxi' the Robot that Supports Nurses | Diligent Robotics.* https://www.youtube.com/watch?v=Pdm0hix7OiI

   Medium. (2023). The future of nursing: Can robots and AI step into the shoes of human nurses? https://drdiplextechnomad.medium.com/the-future-of-nursing-can-robots-and-ai-step-into-the-shoes-of-human-nurses-ef82897f86ec

2. Advanced technology for nursing education:
   American Nurses Foundation. (n.d.). *Disrupting nursing education with XR, AI and ML*. https://www.nursingworld.org/foundation/rninitiative/practice-ready-nurse-graduates/disrupting-nursing-education-with-xr-ai-and-ml

3. Online Learning Consortium is a consortium of online educators who are "dedicated to advancing quality digital teaching and learning experiences designed to reach and engage the modern learner—anyone, anywhere, anytime.": https://onlinelearningconsortium.org

REFERENCES

American Nurses Foundation. (2024a). *Disrupting nursing education with XR, AI and ML*. https://www.nursingworld.org/foundation/rninitiative/practice-ready-nurse-graduates/disrupting-nursing-education-with-xr-ai-and-ml

American Nurses Foundation. (2024b). *Driving nursing outcomes through robotics*. https://www.nursingworld.org/foundation/rninitiative/technology-enabled-nursing-practice/driving-nursing-outcomes-through-robotics

Arcega, J., Autman, I., De Guzman, B., Isidienu, L., Olivar, J., O'Neal, M., & Surdilla, B. (2020). The human touch: Is modern technology decreasing the value of humanity in patient care? *Critical Care Nursing Quarterly, 43*(3), 294–302. https://doi.org/10.1097/CNQ.0000000000000314

Coursera. (2024). *4 types of AI: getting to know artificial intelligence*. https://www.coursera.org/articles/types-of-ai

Diligent Robotics. (2023, September). LinkedIn. https://www.linkedin.com/posts/diligent-robotics_100-moxi-robots-to-be-in-30-hospitals-by-activity-7111043670975418368-SVQv/

Emmy, M. (2023). *The future of e-learning: trends and predictions for 2023 and beyond*. eLearning Industry. https://elearningindustry.com/future-of-elearning-trends-and-predictions-for-2023-and-beyond

Evanick, J. (2023, June 27). *Immersive learning: How virtual and augmented reality are transforming higher education*. eLearning Industry. https://elearningindustry.com/immersive-learning-how-virtual-and-augmented-reality-transforming-higher-education

Frith, K. H. (2021). Robots are promising innovations for nursing practice. *Nursing Education Perspectives (Wolters Kluwer Health), 42*(6), 383. https://doi-org/10.1097/01.NEP.0000000000000901

Google (2023). Glass *enterprise edition 2 Announcement* FAQ. https://support.google.com/glass-enterprise/customer/answer/13417888?sjid=13369235504290142161-NC

Healthcare Dive. (2024). *Trends in telehealth: The future of virtual care*. https://www.healthcaredive.com/spons/trends-in-telehealth-the-future-of-virtual-care/709544/

Henry, J. (2022, December 23). Immersive learning design today: Best practices. *eLearning Industry*. https://elearningindustry.com/immersive-learning-design-today-best-practices

IBM. (n.d.) *What is artificial intelligence (AI)?* https://www.ibm.com/topics/artificial-intelligence

IBM. (2023). *Understanding the different types of artificial intelligence*. https://www.ibm.com/blog/understanding-the-different-types-of-artificial-intelligence

Johnson, E., & Carrington, J. M. (2023). Revisiting the nursing metaparadigm: Acknowledging technology as foundational to progressing nursing knowledge. *Nursing Inquiry, 30*(1), 1–6. https://doi.org/10.1111/nin.12502

Korn, J. (2023, March 16). *Google will stop selling Glass as it looks to cut costs.* CNN Business. https://www.cnn.com/2023/03/16/tech/google-glass-gone/index.html

Mda Training. (2023). *The future of digital learning: 7 trends to watch in 2024.* LinkedIn. https://www.linkedin.com/pulse/future-digital-learning-7-trends-watch-2024-mda-training-sbb6f/

Pitts, N. (2023, September 6). How to be conspicuously human in the online classroom. *Faculty Focus.* https://www.facultyfocus.com/articles/online-education/online-course-delivery-and-instruction/how-to-be-conspicuously-human-in-the-online-classroom/

Registered Nurses Association of Ontario. (2020). Nursing and compassionate care in the age of artificial intelligence: Engaging the emerging future. *AMS Healthcare.* 2–42. https://www.ams-inc.on.ca/resource/nursing-and-compassionate-care-in-the-age-of-artificial-intelligence/

Rony, M. K. K., Kayesh, I., Bala, S. D., Akter, F., & Parvin, M. R. (2024). Artificial intelligence in future nursing care: Exploring perspectives of nursing professionals—A descriptive qualitative study. *Heliyon, 10*(4), e25718. https://doi.org/10.1016/j.heliyon.2024.e25718

Rubeis, G. (2021). Guardians of humanity? The challenges of nursing practice in the digital age. *Nursing Philosophy,* 22, e12331. https://doi.org/10.1111/nup.12331

Siwicki, B. (2017). *86% of healthcare companies use some form of AI.* Healthcare IT News. https://www.healthcareitnews.com/news/86-healthcare-companies-use-some-form-ai

Spilka, D. (2023, May 8). *How VR and AR are revolutionizing eLearning for learners of all ages.* eLearning Industries. https://elearningindustry.com/how-vr-and-ar-are-revolutionizing-elearning-for-learners-of-all-ages

Stokes, F., & Palmer, A. (2020). Artificial intelligence and robotics in nursing: Ethics of caring as a guide to dividing tasks between AI and humans. *Nursing Philosophy, 21*(4), 1–9. https://doi.org/10.1111/nup.12306

Towards Healthcare. (2022). *AR and VR in healthcare market size envisioned at USD 13.74 billion by 2032.* https://www.towardshealthcare.com/insights/augmented-and-virtual-reality-in-healthcare-market

Credits

Index

www.ingramcontent.com/pod-product-compliance
Ingram Content Group UK Ltd.
Pitfield, Milton Keynes, MK11 3LW, UK
UKHW021831270726
14058UKWH00001B/89